AF597515

Advances in Computer Vision and Pattern Recognition

For other titles published in this series, go to
www.springer.com/series/4205

Ananda S. Chowdhury · Suchendra M. Bhandarkar

Computer Vision-Guided Virtual Craniofacial Surgery

A Graph-Theoretic and Statistical Perspective

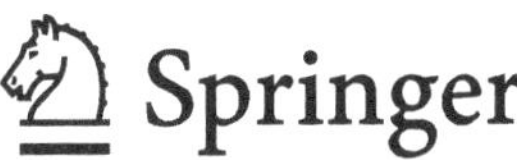

Dr. Ananda S. Chowdhury
Department of Electronics &
Telecommunication Engineering
Jadavpur University
188 Raja S.C. Malik Road
700032 Kolkata, West Bengal
India
ananda.chowdhury@gmail.com

Prof. Suchendra M. Bhandarkar
Department of Computer Science
The University of Georgia
Boyd Graduate Studies Research Center
Room 415
30602-7404 Athens, GA
USA
suchi@cs.uga.edu

Series Editors
Professor Sameer Singh, PhD
Research School of Informatics
Loughborough University
Loughborough
UK

Dr. Sing Bing Kang
Microsoft Research
Microsoft Corporation
One Microsoft Way
Redmond, WA 98052
USA

ISSN 2191-6586
ISBN 978-0-85729-295-7 e-ISBN 978-0-85729-296-4
DOI 10.1007/978-0-85729-296-4
Springer London Dordrecht Heidelberg New York

British Library Cataloguing in Publication Data
A catalogue record for this book is available from the British Library

Library of Congress Control Number: 2011923551

Cover design: deblik

Printed on acid-free paper

Springer is part of Springer Science+Business Media (www.springer.com)

To my wife Anindita
– Ananda S. Chowdhury

To my wife Swati, son Pranav, and daughter Asha
– Suchendra M. Bhandarkar

Foreword

An ancient mariner on the open seas had to know where he is before he could navigate to where he had to go. A surgeon, through training and experience, gains a mental image of what that "map" should be. It is called surgical anatomy. This is possible because for the most part, the human anatomy, at the large-scale level (1 cm to 10 cm, for example), is not exceedingly variable. However, to know the precise location of the surgery, dissection is needed to allow either direct visualization or palpation of the particular anatomic structures. Often, such dissection is associated with disruption of normal tissues, interruption of blood supply, prolonging the magnitude of surgery, increasing the risk of potential complications, and lengthening the post-operative convalescence. In recent times, Computer Tomography (CT) and Magnetic Resonance Imaging (MRI) have allowed the surgeon to see this surgical map at a level of detail and precision not previously possible. Recent advances in both scanning instruments and supporting software have transitioned their impact from merely outside the operating room to inside the surgical theater, making intraoperative 3D imaging a reality.

However, most of the existing intraoperative navigation devices are still bulky, time-consuming to use, and increase the potential for contaminating the sterile operative field. Given that the cost per minute in the operating room continues to sky rocket, the more work that can be done before entering the operating room, the more effective and efficient the surgeon can be. This monograph details a collaborative research endeavor over the past five years at the University of Georgia and the Medical College of Georgia in designing a software system that can reconstitute broken bones *in silico*, either through a graphical user interface or in an automated fashion from fracture detection to fracture reduction—a process where the displaced bone fragments are returned to where they should be. The sizes and shapes of the fractured bone(s) and the shape of the *in silico* reconstruction can be obtained and then linked to CAD–CAM devices. Reconstruction plates can then be shaped to fit precisely the individual anatomy, and the optimal lengths, orientations, and locations of the various screws can be determined. Armed with this customized fixation hardware, a surgeon can drastically reduce the time needed in the operating room and, as long as an accurate fiduciary transfer is made, achieve an accurate reduction and fixation of the fractures with significantly less extensive dissection. This approach improves the current state-of-the-art by increasing accuracy, decreasing cost, and reducing both the operative trauma and the risk of operative and postoperative complications to the patient.

As a practicing plastic surgeon, I can recall many times when I wished I had such a software system at my disposal. It was largely on account of this pressing need that we embarked, some six years ago, upon this research endeavor. Having the ability to detect and manipulate the fracture fragments, and return them to their preinjury state *in silico* will allow the surgeons to obtain a more accurate reduction and reconstruction with less extensive dissection. The end result is a much shorter operating time and significantly improved surgical outcome. This monograph is the culminating achievement of the sustained efforts of many people, especially Dr. Ananda Chowdhury, then a Ph.D. candidate at the University of Georgia, and my dear friend, Dr. Suchendra Bhandarkar, Ananda's doctoral research advisor. It is through such collaborative work that we can realize significant, high-impact advances that contribute to the surgical treatment of patients with cranio-maxillofacial fractures.

Jack C. Yu, DMD, MD, MS Ed, FACS, FADI
Milford B. Hatcher Professor of Surgery
and Chief
Section of Plastic Surgery
School of Medicine
Medical College of Georgia
Augusta, GA, USA

Preface

The monograph deals with an important application of computer vision and pattern recognition in the area of medical science, more specifically reconstructive craniofacial surgery. Craniofacial fractures are encountered very frequently in today's fast-paced society; the major causes being gunshot wounds, motor vehicle accidents, and sports-related injuries. Surgical reconstruction is challenging because the surgeons in the operating room have to register the broken bone fragments accurately and under severe time constraints. Within the broad class of craniofacial fractures, the emphasis in this monograph is on mandibular fractures since the mandible is often unprotected and exposed making it especially vulnerable to accidents and injuries. A typical input to a computer vision-based system for virtual craniofacial surgery is a sequence of Computed Tomography (CT) images of a fractured human mandible. The detection of fractures in CT images, the other integral component of reconstructive craniofacial surgery, is often difficult because of the complexity of the fracture patterns, missing data, image intensity inhomogeneities, and presence of noise and undesired artifacts.

A formal treatment of computer vision-guided craniofacial surgery entails the solving of two broad classes of problems, i.e., computer-aided fracture detection and virtual reconstruction, both of which raise several important theoretical and practical issues. From a theoretical standpoint, the monograph discusses several traditional topics in computer vision and pattern recognition such as image registration, image reconstruction, combinatorial pattern matching, and detection of salient points and regions in an image. Several useful algorithms and concepts from two traditionally diverse disciplines, namely, graph theory and statistics are seen to be applicable in this context. The relevant topics from graph theory include maximum-weight graph matching, maximum-cardinality minimum-weight matching for a bipartite graph, maximum-flow minimum-cut determination in a flow graph, and construction of automorphs of a cycle graph. The monograph demonstrates how the above graph-theoretic algorithms can be applied to solve some important problems in computer vision and pattern recognition that pertain to virtual reconstructive craniofacial surgery. The various statistical techniques brought to bear include Markov random fields, hierarchical Bayesian restoration, Gibbs sampling, and Bayesian inference.

We show how these sophisticated statistical methods can solve very important problems in the area of virtual reconstructive craniofacial surgery; problems which are of general interest to the broader computer vision and pattern recognition community as well.

From a practical application-oriented viewpoint, we focus, in this monograph, on a highly relevant biomedical problem, i.e., reconstructive craniofacial surgery. The two integral components of any reconstructive surgery, namely, the detection and localization of fractures, and the subsequent reconstruction from the broken bone fragments, are addressed in depth. The proposed solutions for virtual craniofacial reconstruction and computer-aided fracture detection are aimed principally at increasing significantly the current extent of automation in reconstructive craniofacial surgery. However, the proposed solutions have the inherent potential to tackle similar problems in related fields such as radiology, orthopedic surgery, and histopathology.

The monograph consists of four parts that develop the subject matter in a logically coherent manner. Part I of the monograph contains three chapters which provide a broad overview of the subject and the necessary theoretical foundations. In Chap. 1, we discuss in detail, the overall importance of the proposed work. In Chap. 2, we present some important concepts and algorithms from graph theory, which include graph matching, graph isomorphism, graph automorphism, and network flows. In Chap. 3, we discuss some basic and advanced statistical concepts such as probability, inference, Bayesian statistics, and random fields. Suitable illustrations and examples are used in both Chaps. 2 and 3 to familiarize a general reader with these important concepts. The materials covered in Chaps. 2 and 3 are used extensively in the remainder of the monograph to solve the problems of virtual reconstruction and computer-aided fracture detection.

Part II of the monograph, consisting of Chaps. 4 and 5, is dedicated to virtual craniofacial reconstruction. Chapter 4 is devoted to the different aspects of virtual craniofacial reconstruction in the presence of a single fracture. In this chapter, we discuss various surface matching techniques such as the Iterative Closest Point (ICP) algorithm and the Data Aligned Rigidity Constrained Exhaustive Search (DARCES) algorithm. In addition, we describe how the incorporation of knowledge of bilateral symmetry, biomechanical stability, and suitable modeling of fracture surface irregularity can improve the overall reconstruction accuracy. The Maximum Cardinality Minimum Weight Bipartite Graph Matching algorithm, relevant concepts from Graph Automorphism, Fuzzy set-theoretic modeling, and extraction of mean and Gaussian curvature values from the fracture surfaces are applied at various stages of the reconstruction process. In Chap. 5, the problem of virtual craniofacial reconstruction in the presence of multiple fractures is investigated. This problem is shown to resemble that of assembly of a complex 3D jigsaw puzzle from individual pieces. Thus, the nature of the problem of virtual multifracture reconstruction is shown to be combinatorial in terms of the number of reconstruction options with a worst-case exponential-time algorithmic complexity. In an alternative formulation, this problem is modeled as one of maximum weight graph matching, which has a worst-case polynomial-time algorithmic complexity.

Part III of the monograph consists of three chapters; Chaps. 6, 7, and 8, which focus on the problem of computer-aided fracture detection. In Chap. 6, we present techniques for detecting surface points on major or well-displaced fractures, which denote situations where the broken bone fragments exhibit noticeable relative displacements. Points of high surface curvature are first detected on potential fracture surfaces in individual CT image slices. A Kalman filter formulation, within a Bayesian inference paradigm, is subsequently used to remove spurious surface points. Chapter 7 discusses the detection of hairline or minor fractures which arise in situations where the broken bone fragments are not visibly out of alignment. A hierarchical Bayesian restoration framework is formulated to detect the hairline fracture and also generate the target pattern which simulates the end result of the bone healing process. We model the fracture as a local stochastic degradation of a hypothetical intact mandible and show how a Markov random field (MRF), incorporated within a hierarchical Bayesian framework, can be used to solve the problem. In Chap. 8, in an alternative formulation, a hairline or minor fracture is modeled as a minimum cut in an appropriately weighted flow network. The classical Ford–Fulkerson algorithm is employed to determine the minimum cut in the aforementioned flow network. Each all of the five chapters on virtual craniofacial reconstruction and computer-aided fracture detection discuss a specific problem and are organized in the following manner:

1. Each chapter starts with a section that introduces and motivates the specific problem.
2. Each chapter discusses the related work for the specific problem and highlights the novelty of the proposed solution.
3. Each chapter presents the theoretical foundations underlying the proposed solution.
4. Each chapter includes a section of experimental results with in-depth analysis.
5. Each chapter contains a conclusion and future work section for the specific problem.

Part IV of the monograph consists of a single chapter. In this final chapter (Chap. 9), we summarize our overall contributions and present a design for a Graphical User Interface (GUI) in which the different methods for virtual craniofacial reconstruction and computer-aided fracture detection are integrated. A section on future research directions is also included. This section, in contrast to the *Conclusions and Future Work* section at the end of each of the Chaps. 4–9 (which focus on a specific problem discussed in that chapter), provides a holistic view of the general directions for future research work in the broader area of computer vision-guided virtual surgery.

The monograph is meant to address a fairly diverse audience including researchers, university faculty, graduate students, and clinical practitioners such as plastic surgeons, orthopedic surgeons, and radiologists. Researchers and graduate students in various diverse disciplines such as computer science, electrical engineering, biomedical engineering, and statistics would find the topics covered in this monograph to be very useful. The formal and elegant modeling of some very general problems in the area of computer vision and pattern recognition by means of graph theory and statistics would be attractive to researchers and graduate students in computer science, computer engineering, and electrical engineering. The monograph can be used in a one-semester graduate-level course dealing with special topics in computer vision as part of a graduate curriculum in a computer science, computer engineering, or electrical engineering department. Since the monograph presents an elaborate treatise on a relevant biomedical problem, it would be of potential interest to researchers and graduate students in biomedical engineering as well. Researchers and graduate students in statistics with interest in statistical pattern recognition would also find several of the topics, covered in this monograph, very useful. Practicing surgeons in the field of reconstructive craniofacial surgery in particular, and orthopedic surgery in general, and radiologists interested in computer-aided detection of craniofacial fractures in CT scans would also benefit greatly from the research described in the monograph.

We sincerely acknowledge the help and advice of many people in preparing this monograph. We appreciate the strong encouragement of Prof. Sameer Singh and Dr. Sing Bing Kang, the series editors of the "Advances in Computer Vision and Pattern Recognition" monograph series published by Springer. We express our sincere thanks to Dr. Wayne Wheeler, the managing editor for this Springer monograph series, for his useful guidance, and to Mr. Simon Rees and Ms. Catherine Brett for their editorial help. We owe a debt of gratitude to Prof. Robert W. Robinson, Dr. Jack C. Yu, Prof. Gauri S. Datta, Dr. Archan Bhattachraya, Ms. Yarong Tang, Prof. Hamid R. Arabnia, Prof. Ernest W. Tollner, Dr. Edmond Ritter, Dr. Ramon Figueroa, and Prof. Amit Konar for their involvement in the research, described in this monograph, at various stages. Ananda S. Chowdhury was a doctoral student under the supervision of Prof. Suchendra M. Bhandarkar in the Department of Computer Science at the University of Georgia, Athens, Georgia, when the research described in the monograph was carried out. The writing of this monograph began when Dr. Chowdhury was working with Dr. Ronald M. Summers in the Department of Radiology and Imaging Sciences at the National Institutes of Health, Bethesda, Maryland, as a postdoctoral fellow. The monograph was eventually completed after Dr. Chowdhury joined the Department of Electronics and Telecommunication Engineering at Jadavpur University, Kolkata, India, as a faculty member. Dr. Ananda S. Chowdhury deeply appreciates the constant support and encouragement of his parents Dr. Subarna Chowdhury and Prof. Satyabrata Chowdhury, his wife Anindita, and his brother Subha during the course of this research and the writing of the monograph. Prof. Suchendra M. Bhandarkar would like to express his deepest gratitude to his wife Swati, son Pranav, and daughter Asha for their constant encouragement, patience, and understanding during the writing of this monograph. This research work was supported in part by research grants from the Biomedical and Health Sciences Institute (BHSI), Faculty of Engineering (FE), and the University of Georgia Research Foundation (UGARF) at the University of Georgia, Athens, Georgia.

Bethesda, MD, USA
Kolkata, India
Athens, GA, USA

Ananda S. Chowdhury

Suchendra M. Bhandarkar

Contents

List of Figures

List of Tables

Part I
Overview and Foundations

Chapter 1
Introduction

This monograph is devoted to an in-depth exposition of the various issues that arise in virtual reconstructive craniofacial surgery and is written from a graph-theoretic and statistical perspective. We discuss some sophisticated techniques from computer vision, graph theory, and statistics and demonstrate how they can be employed to address the various challenging problems that arise in virtual reconstructive craniofacial surgery. The solutions presented here are quite general in their scope and applicability. Consequently, they can be easily applied to tackle similar problems that arise in related areas such as reconstructive orthopedic surgery and seemingly unrelated areas such as archeology, where ancient artifacts such as pottery need to be virtually reconstructed from unearthed broken pieces. This will be more evident in the discussion of the individual problems in the later chapters of the monograph. In this chapter, we first describe the anatomy of craniofacial fractures. Next, we discuss the state-of-the-art in the field of virtual reconstructive craniofacial surgery. Then, we highlight the importance of our contributions. We end this chapter by outlining the organization of this monograph.

1.1 Craniofacial Fractures

Craniofacial fractures are encountered very frequently in today's fast-paced modern society, the principal causes being motor vehicle accidents and sports-related injuries [1]. In addition, fractures resulting from craniofacial injuries are greatly prevalent in battlefield situations and occur primarily due to gunshot and shrapnel wounds. The craniofacial skeleton is usually less protected than other parts of the human anatomy, even with full-body armor or any other form of protective clothing, leading to such a large incidence of craniofacial fractures. Ogundare et al. [2], in their research, illustrated that the observed craniofacial fracture patterns sometimes imply the existence of a single fracture and, in some other cases, a combination of single fractures. As shown by Zahl et al. [3], the cost of surgery becomes prohibitive, not to mention the increased operative and post-operative risk to the patient, with

A.S. Chowdhury, S.M. Bhandarkar, *Computer Vision-Guided Virtual Craniofacial Surgery*, Advances in Computer Vision and Pattern Recognition,
DOI 10.1007/978-0-85729-296-4_1,

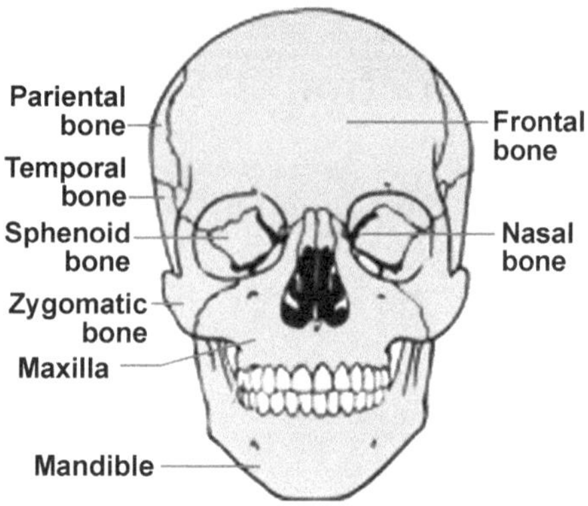

Fig. 1.1 Frontal view of craniofacial skeleton. Source: American Medical Association. All rights reserved

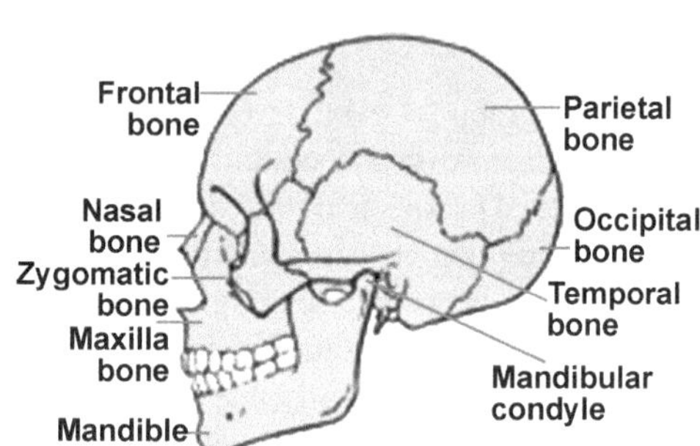

Fig. 1.2 Side view of craniofacial skeleton. Source: American Medical Association. All rights reserved

the increased operating time necessary to ensure an accurate reconstruction. This is especially true in complex trauma situations that involve multiple fractures.

Bone is a unique structure found only among members of the Phylum Chordata. It is the only living material in the entire animal kingdom that possesses a compressive modulus in the range of 1.0 N/m^2 to 1.0×10^{10} N/m^2 with a volumetric range from 10^{-9} m^3 to 10 m^3. Bone is the rigid element in the body which resists deformation, allows for transmission of forces, and protects the internal organs. The craniofacial skeleton consists of high stress-bearing buttresses and low stress-bearing curve planes. Figures 1.1 and 1.2 show two different views of the craniofacial anatomy. Figure 1.1 shows the frontal view of the craniofacial skeleton, whereas Fig. 1.2 illustrates the side view of the same. When external loads are applied, the craniofacial skeleton undergoes strain. When the strain exceeds the ultimate strain limit, about 1.0×10^4 microstrains, failure occurs [4]. The resulting loss of spatial continuity in the craniofacial skeleton is termed clinically as *fracture* which causes pain, disfigurement, and functional impairment due to the disruption of force transmission. However, unlike any man-made material, bone, being living tissue, is capable of healing. For this healing to occur, there are two cardinal requirements, sufficient blood supply and relative stability.

In clinical treatment of fractures, the proper realignment of the bone fragments must be achieved *prior* to fracture healing. Improper realignment of the fragments results in *malunion*. The younger the individual, the more robust the healing and remodeling potential and thus better the tolerance to malunion. In the case of the

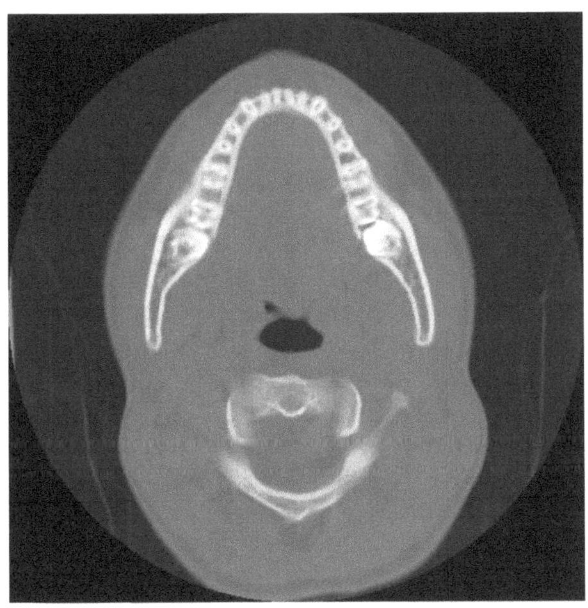

Fig. 1.3 CT scan of an intact mandible

fracture of the upper and lower jaws, an inherent dilemma exists. Since the maxilla (upper jaw) and mandible (lower jaw) house the 32 permanent teeth, which must fit precisely in a particular orientation known as the *position of intercuspation*, malunion is very poorly tolerated. In order to prevent malunion, extensive dissection must be done to visualize all the fractures. However, the resulting stripping of the periosteum inevitably reduces the amount of blood flow to the bone fragments. Due to the three-dimensional (3D) geometry of the masticatory system, an angular malalignment of 1° in the anterior region of the mandible typically results in an 8–10-mm transverse displacement in the area of the secondary molars. This transverse displacement severely disrupts the intercuspation and constitutes a dreaded postoperative condition known as *malocclusion*. The two condyles serve as anatomical landmarks for any given mandible. The side view of the craniofacial skeleton in Fig. 1.2 shows one of the condyles. In some extreme cases of malocclusion, the mandibular width can be so altered that the condyles are no longer within the glenoid fossas of the temporal mandibular joints thus severely disrupting the masticatory function.

A transverse Computed Tomography (CT) scan of an intact mandible is shown in Fig. 1.3. The CT scan protocol is typically set by the radiologist. In the present work, both, the fine *thin-cut protocol* comprising of CT image slices taken 1 mm apart and the quick *coarse-cut protocol* comprising of CT image slices taken 3–5 mm apart are used. The thin-cut protocol is employed for examining detailed bone structure. However, if the condition of a patient becomes unstable, e.g., due to extensive haemorrhaging in the cranial cavity, it is imperative that the CT scan be performed and the patient transported from the CT scanner room to the operating

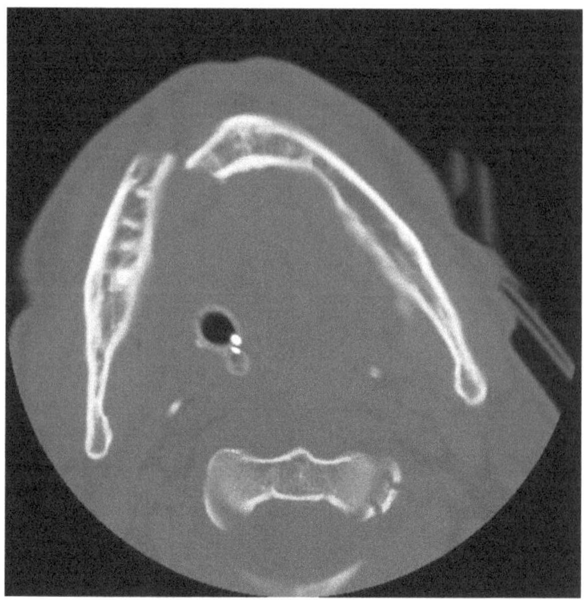

Fig. 1.4 CT scan of a mandible with a major fracture

room as soon as possible. The quick coarse-cut protocol is more appropriate in such situations.

As seen in Fig. 1.3, the intensity of the mandible in the CT image slice is bright on account of its bony structure. Also, the shape of the mandible is observed to be parabolic, i.e., similar to that of a horse shoe. On the other hand, the soft tissue and other artifacts are observed to exhibit a lower intensity in the CT image slice compared to the mandible. In Fig. 1.4, we show an image slice from a CT scan of a mandible with a major or well-displaced fracture which is observed to lie near the middle portion of the mandible. Note that the two broken bone fragments exhibit noticeable relative displacement in this case. In Fig. 1.5, we show an image slice from a CT scan of a phantom mandible with a similar major fracture. The phantom is essentially a high-quality radio-opaque plastic model of human skull. Working with phantoms allows one to compare the results of the computer-aided reconstruction with the CT scan data of the intact phantom (i.e., prior to fracture). Note that the prefracture CT scan data is typically not available in real craniofacial trauma cases.

The prefracture CT scan of the phantom is generated by putting it through the CT scanner using the thin-cut protocol. The skull is then fractured by applying a compressive force to the gonial angle, i.e., the angle formed by the intersection of the corpus of the mandible and the ascending mandibular ramus. The resulting bone fragments are then held in the desired displaced position to simulate the displacement of bone fragments in real facial fractures. This construct is then subject to a CT scan using the same thin-cut protocol. The CT image slices in Figs. 1.6 and 1.7 are from CT scans of two mandibles with a minor or hairline fracture. In Fig. 1.6, a small rectangle shows the hairline fracture in the bottom-left portion of

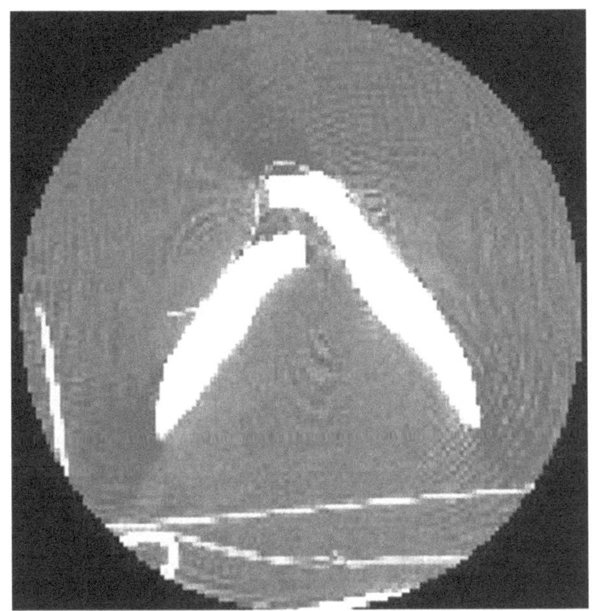

Fig. 1.5 CT scan of a phantom mandible with a major fracture

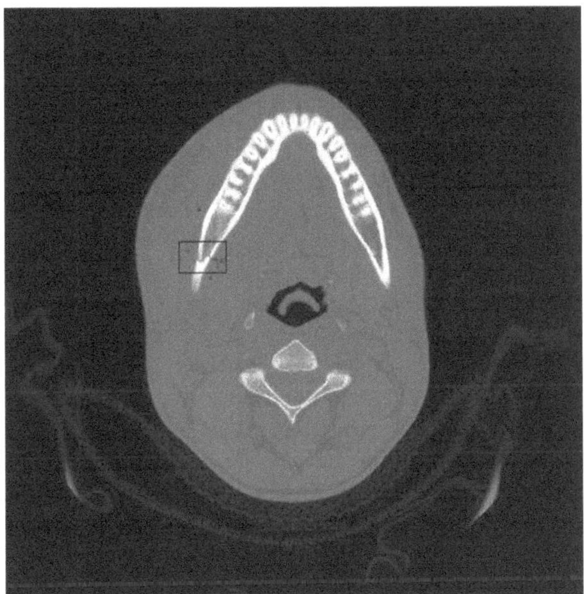

Fig. 1.6 CT scan of a mandible with a hairline fracture

the mandible. Similarly, a small rectangle in Fig. 1.7 indicates that the hairline fracture lies in the top-right portion of the mandible. In the two hairline fractures shown above, the broken bone fragments are observed to suffer a visually insignificant displacement relative to each other.

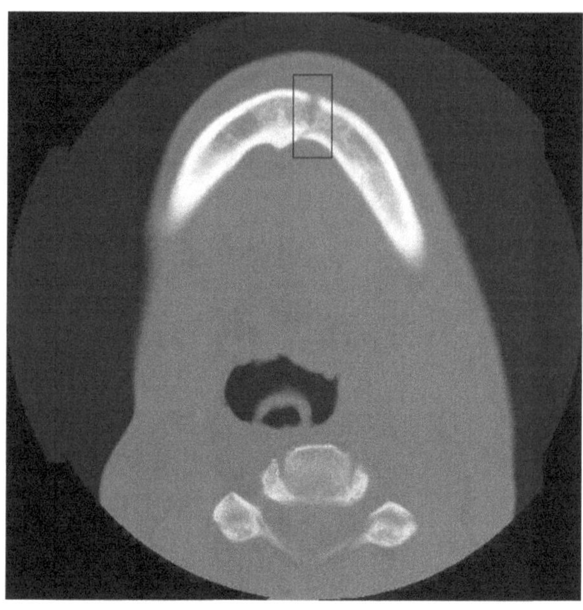

Fig. 1.7 CT scan of another mandible with a hairline fracture

1.2 State-of-the-Art Virtual Craniofacial Surgery

While there exists recent work published in the literature dealing with simulation of mandibular fractures [5, 6], and simulation of dental implantalogy [7] there is little reported, in recent years, by way of automated computer-aided surgical reconstruction of the craniofacial skeleton and detection of craniofacial fractures. There has been some recent progress in the design of thoracolumbosacral orthosis braces using Computed Tomography (CT) and Magnetic Resonance (MR) images of the spinal region for postoperative patients needing back correction and support [8]. Computer-aided surgical planning has also been explored in the context of orthopedic surgery [9–11] and rhinoplasty [12]. Previous research in surgical planning using computer visualization in the context of oral, maxillofacial, craniofacial, orthodontic, or orthognathic surgery includes the works of Ayoub et al. [13], Gerbo et al. [14], and Hassfeld et al. [15]. Patel et al. [16] have examined the issues involved in computer-assisted craniofacial surgical planning and simulation using CT, computer visualization, and graphical simulation techniques. They have discussed a quantitative assessment of craniofacial surgical simulation where the surgical procedures are carried out on cadavers, both in physical reality and virtual reality (*in silico*). The CT reconstruction after the physical (i.e., actual) surgery is compared with that resulting from the virtual surgery using volume registration methods and quantitative error metrics. The surgical procedures are performed on the cranial region and not the mandibular region which is the focus of this monograph.

Verstreken et al. [17] have discussed a preoperative planning system for oral implant surgery which takes as input CT images of the upper and lower jaws. Hilger et al. [18] have investigated the modeling of craniofacial bone growth using generative models for the temporal shape and size of the human mandible that are mapped into Procrustes tangent space. Cevidanes et al. [19] have described image processing methods for the computation of morphometric changes associated with jaw surgery, precisely locating jaw displacements and quantitatively describing the vectors of displacement. Enciso et al. [20] and Mollemans et al. [21] have examined issues pertaining to soft-tissue modeling and simulation of jaw motion in the context of virtual craniofacial surgery. The multidisciplinary Imaging Technology Group (ITG) at the University of Illinois, Urbana-Champaign has investigated an alternative approach to bone replacement in the context of reconstructive craniofacial surgery [22]. An integrated workflow from the surgeon to the 3D craniofacial modeler to the implant fabricator has been developed that yields a perfectly fitting custom implant. The feasibility of this approach in a real clinical setting has also been demonstrated. However, the focus of this project has been on the material science aspect of implant fabrication rather than on automation of the craniofacial reconstruction using machine vision and machine learning techniques.

A team of researchers at the Stanford University Medical Center has investigated the development of a virtual reality environment for surgical planning in the context of craniofacial and mandibular reconstruction [23]. A realistic 3D virtual environment that models the soft tissue and skeletal structure from CT scans of the patient has been developed. The virtual reality surgical environment has been designed to allow the surgeon to better understand the problem and perform the proposed procedure. This system was tested on a group of select patients with difficult congenital malformations. However, the system has been designed to be purely interactive with no automation of the craniofacial reconstruction procedures using machine vision and machine learning techniques. Last but not the least, Ahmed et al. [24] have presented an approach for 3D reconstruction of the human jaw from a sequence of intra-oral images taken by a CCD camera mounted on the stylus of a hand-held digitizer that a surgeon can use to scan the inside of a patient's mouth. A novel space carving algorithm is used to perform shape recovery for jaw reconstruction. The focus of the work is on 3D jaw reconstruction for the purpose of orthodontics with the goal of replacing the cumbersome and expensive process of creating dental casts or imprints. The problem of computer-aided fracture detection and virtual craniofacial reconstruction, however, is not addressed.

An in-depth review of the state-of-the-art has revealed the relative paucity of existing work on computer-aided virtual craniofacial reconstruction and fracture detection. This reinforces our thesis that the research presented in the monograph is at the cutting edge of computer-assisted surgical planning, especially in the area of reconstructive craniofacial surgery.

1.3 The Importance of Computer-Assisted Surgical Planning

A computer-integrated orthopedic system, called FRACAS, was designed by Joskowicz et al. for assisting surgeons to perform long bone surgery in the last decade [25]. A recent report by the American Medical Association has predicted that major breakthroughs in the field of surgery in the first half of the 21st century will result from surgical robotization and automation [26]. It is expected that advances in computer-assisted surgery would allow surgeons to do what is currently infeasible, and also to do it with greater efficiency and precision. In image-guided surgery, multimodal preoperative images are registered to each other and to the patient and used to track the surgical instruments in real time during the procedure. An interactive display of a realistic 3D model of the operative volume is used to guide the surgeon in real time [27].

Intraoperative imaging and 3D visualization have been successfully deployed for brain tumor surgery where the goal is careful removal of tumor tissue without damaging the adjacent functionally critical structures. Image-guided surgery is used to perform tasks like lesion detection and finding the anatomical relationships of a tumor tissue with adjacent functionally critical structures [28]. A related concept under the broad spectrum of computer-assisted surgical planning, which has gained popularity over the past few years, is image-guided therapy [29]. Image-guided therapy combines surface-based visualization with volumetric information. By merging images from different modalities, pathologic changes and their anatomic locations are integrated within the same framework under this new approach. An interesting application of image-guided therapy can be found in pediatric interventional radiology [30].

The overarching goal of the research presented in this monograph is to develop an enabling technology that leverages the advances in computer vision, graph theory, and statistics for the purpose of virtual (*in silico*) craniofacial reconstructive surgery. The intended final outcome is an interactive graphical software that could be used as a decision support system for *presurgical planning* as opposed to real-time surgical guidance. The input to the software is a series of CT images showing a fractured craniofacial skeleton. The output of the software is a virtual reconstruction of the craniofacial skeleton along with proper detection of the fracture(s). An enhanced version of the software would also allow for the automated or semi-automated design and affixation of appropriate prostheses such as titanium miniplates, screws, grafts, and implants. The same graphical software, with little modification, could also be used by medical students and surgery residents as an interactive training tool. The software would allow the user to experiment with virtual craniofacial reconstruction strategies using a variety of prostheses *in silico*. The research described in this monograph would constitute the necessary preliminary step toward defect-directed bone substitution by tissue-engineered constructs. In future, the surgical planning software could be potentially interfaced with a telerobotic system that could allow a surgeon to perform the surgery remotely.

The principal advantages of the research described in this monograph include:

1. enabling the plastic surgeon to visualize the end product, i.e., the reconstructed jaw, before performing the actual surgery,
2. automated or semi-automated detection of fractures from X-ray or CT images in the possible presence of image intensity inhomogeneities and noise,
3. automated or semi-automated means of virtual (*in silico*) craniofacial reconstruction,

4. automated or semi-automated means for the design and affixation of the necessary prostheses such as titanium miniplates, screws, grafts, and implants,
5. increased accuracy of the post-surgical craniofacial reconstruction, and
6. a several-fold reduction in the time and effort required for the actual surgery in the operating room; this would be especially true in complex craniofacial trauma cases with multiple fractures.

On successful deployment of the research described in this monograph, a patient with severe craniofacial trauma will have CT images of his/her fractured craniofacial skeleton loaded into the presurgical planning system. The system will automatically recognize the fracture surfaces, generate the virtual craniofacial reconstruction by realigning the broken bone fragments *in silico*, and feed the results of the virtual reconstruction to a laser 3D lithographic printer which will generate a reconstructed, life-size polymer-epoxy model of the craniofacial skeleton. The prostheses manufacturers, using this epoxy model, will be able to machine the miniplates to best brace the fractures, select screws of the optimum size and length, and select the positions on the model where the screws can be placed in an anatomically safe and biomechanically sound manner. Likewise, appropriate grafts and implants will be designed to account for missing bone fragments. Alternatively, the positions, shapes, and dimensions of the miniplates, screws, grafts, and implants can be determined automatically by the system from the virtual craniofacial reconstruction. The entire construct will be sent back to the surgeon in the operating room, and the surgery will be carried out in a much shorter time frame with vastly improved accuracy. In addition, this technology will potentially allow the prostheses and other fixation devices to be deployed using endoscopic or minimally invasive surgical procedures.

The successful deployment of the research described in this monograph will also have a significant economic impact on the costs of reconstructive craniofacial surgery. The current operating room costs are approximately $20 per minute. If the actual time required in miniplate and screw selection, miniplate adaptation, and graft or implant customization during the surgery can be reduced by 30 minutes per miniplate, graft, or implant, then this would translate to savings of $1,200 per case assuming that two miniplates, grafts, or implants are deployed per case on average. If the improved accuracy reduces one reoperation or additional operation in 5 cases that would translate to an additional savings of $1,500 per case, assuming that each case costs about $7,500. Thus, the total potential direct operative savings will be $2,700 per case on average. Not including the indirect benefits that accrue from reduced length of hospital stay, earlier return to normal life and reduced occurrence of postoperative complications, the potential total direct operative savings can be as high as 27 million dollars for 100,000 facial trauma patients. With the inclusion of the indirect benefits cited above, the potential savings would be much higher. Thus, the successful completion of the proposed research would result in significant health care cost savings.

In summary, the successful deployment of the research described in this monograph has the potential to save lives, make craniofacial surgery more affordable, and improve the quality of life for patients who have undergone reconstructive craniofacial surgery. Much of the research described in the monograph could also be applied to other forms of reconstructive surgery such as orthopedic surgery. The impact of this research simply cannot be overstated, especially at a time when the United States and several other countries around the world are struggling to find ways and means of reining in the rapidly increasing cost of health care without sacrificing the quality of health care. The research presented in this monograph provides a viable solution to this pressing problem, albeit in the context of reconstructive craniofacial surgery.

1.4 Organization of the Monograph

The monograph is divided into four parts and consists of a total of nine chapters. Part I of the monograph contains three chapters which provide a broad overview of the subject and also the underlying theoretical foundations. In Chap. 1, we discuss in detail the overall importance of the proposed work. In Chap. 2, we present some important concepts and algorithms from graph theory, which include graph matching, graph isomorphism, graph automorphism, and network flows. In Chap. 3, we discuss some basic and advanced statistical concepts such as probability, statistical inference, Bayesian estimation, and random fields. Suitable illustrations and examples are used in both Chaps. 2 and 3 in order to enable a general reader to gain sufficient familiarity with the important concepts contained therein.

Part II of this monograph contains two chapters devoted to the problem of virtual craniofacial reconstruction. Chapters 4 and 5 focus on virtual reconstruction in the presence of a single fracture and multiple fractures, respectively. In Chap. 4, we discuss various surface matching techniques such as the Iterative Closest Point (ICP) algorithm and the Data Aligned Rigidity Constrained Exhaustive Search (DARCES) algorithm. We also show how incorporating the knowledge of anatomical symmetry and biomechanical stability of a human mandible in the reconstruction process improves the overall reconstruction accuracy. The Maximum Cardinality Minimum Weight Bipartite Graph Matching algorithm, relevant concepts from Graph Automorphism, Fuzzy set-theoretic modeling, and extraction of the mean and Gaussian curvature values from the fracture surfaces are employed at various stages of the reconstruction process. In Chap. 5, the problem of virtual craniofacial reconstruction in the presence of multiple fractures is shown to resemble that of automated assembly of a 3D jigsaw puzzle and to have a worst-case exponential-time complexity. In an alternative formulation, the problem of virtual craniofacial reconstruction is modeled as one of maximum-weight graph matching which, in contrast, is shown to have a polynomial-time complexity in the worst case.

Part III of this monograph addresses the problem of computer-aided detection of mandibular fractures. This part contains three chapters (Chaps. 6, 7, and 8), dedicated to various techniques for semi-automatic detection of mandibular fractures. In Chap. 6, we propose a scheme for identification of stable fracture points in well displaced or major fractures in an input CT image sequence. First, a set of candidate fracture points is generated by identifying points of high curvature on the contours of the broken mandibular fragments in the individual 2D CT image slices.

Next, the conventional Kalman filter is modeled as a Bayesian inference problem and used for testing the spatial consistency and stability of the candidate fracture points across the CT image sequence of interest. Chapter 7 discusses a Markov Random Field (MRF)-based hierarchical Bayesian paradigm for detection of hairline or minor fractures and generation of the reconstructed jaw (i.e., target pattern) in such cases. Here, we model the fracture as a local stochastic degradation of a hypothetical intact mandible. In the presence of noise, the detection and subsequent visualization of hairline fractures becomes a clinically challenging task. Furthermore, the decision regarding surgical intervention for this type of fracture is often unclear as a surgeon can choose to rely solely on natural bone healing without any surgical intervention. In addition to aiding in the detection and visualization of the hairline fracture, the generated target pattern depicts how a jaw with a hairline fracture would appear if allowed to heal naturally without explicit surgical intervention. The Bayesian estimation of the mode of the posterior distribution corresponds to the target pattern (i.e., reconstructed jaw), and the differences in intensity between the input data and the MAP estimate at specific pixel locations denote the occurrence and location of a hairline fracture. In Chap. 8, a hairline or minor fracture is modeled alternatively as a minimum cut in an appropriately weighted flow network. Since a hairline fracture can be viewed essentially as a small cut in the bone structure, its detection is modeled as determining the solution to the max-flow min-cut problem in an appropriately constructed flow network. The classical Ford–Fulkerson algorithm is employed to determine a solution to the max-flow min-cut problem and thereby detect a hairline fracture. A minimum cut in the flow network is deemed to correspond to a hairline fracture in the mandibular bone.

The monograph is concluded in Part IV which contains a single chapter that describes the design of a Graphical User Interface (GUI) and summarizes the research accomplishments. In this chapter, the design and functionality of a GUI-driven presurgical planning system, termed as *InsilicoSurgeon*, is illustrated. The GUI for *InsilicoSurgeon* contains many buttons, each designated to execute a specific task. The current version of *InsilicoSurgeon* is designed as a presurgical planning tool for operating surgeons as well as an interactive training tool for medical students and surgery residents. After providing a brief synopsis of our research accomplishments from an interdisciplinary perspective, we conclude the monograph with an outline of future research directions.

Chapter 2
Graph-Theoretic Foundations

In this chapter, we present some important concepts and algorithms from graph theory for the benefit of a general reader. These concepts and algorithms constitute the theoretical underpinnings of a variety of techniques used to solve the various problems that arise in the context of virtual craniofacial surgery. The focus of this chapter is to present the necessary graph-theoretic foundations for the research presented in the remainder of the monograph. The details of the graph-theoretic modeling of specific problems in the context of virtual craniofacial surgery, along with appropriate justifications, will be provided accordingly in the later chapters. This chapter contains an introductory section, followed by three separate sections on graph matching, graph isomorphism, and network flow. We state most of the important theoretical results without proof. The interested reader is referred to reputed textbooks on graph theory such as [31–33], and [34] for a more formal and detailed treatment of the subject.

2.1 Some Basic Terminology

In this section, we discuss some common terminology in graph theory such as the order and the size of a graph, and a walk, a path, and a cycle within a graph following [32]. We also provide the definition of a bipartite graph.

Definition 2.1 A *graph* G is an ordered pair of disjoint sets (V, E) such that E is a subset of the set $V^{(2)}$ of unordered pairs of V. The set V is the set of *vertices*, and E is the set of *edges*.

Definition 2.2 The *order* of G is the number of vertices in G, and the *size* of G is the number of edges in G.

Definition 2.3 A graph $G(V_1 \cup V_2, E)$ is *bipartite* if the two vertex sets V_1 and V_2 are disjoint and every edge in the edge set E joins a vertex in V_1 to a vertex in V_2. The graph G is said to have a bipartition (V_1, V_2).

A.S. Chowdhury, S.M. Bhandarkar, *Computer Vision-Guided Virtual Craniofacial Surgery*, Advances in Computer Vision and Pattern Recognition,
DOI 10.1007/978-0-85729-296-4_2,

Definition 2.4 A *path* P in a graph G is denoted by a sequence of vertices $(v_0, v_1, \ldots, v_n)$ that it connects. In this case, P is said to be a path from v_0 to v_n.

Definition 2.5 A *walk* W in a graph G consists of an alternating sequence of vertices and edges, such as $(v_0, e_1, v_1, e_2, v_2, \ldots, v_{n-1}, e_n, v_n)$, where $e_i = \{v_{i-1}, v_i\}$, $0 < i \leq n$. In this case, W is termed as a $v_0 - v_n$ walk of length n. The difference between a path and a walk is made clear by context in spite of the notational similarity.

Definition 2.6 A graph C_n constitutes a *cycle* of order n if its vertices v_i, $0 < i < n$, are distinct from each other, $n \geq 3$, $v_0 = v_n$, and there exists a $v_0 - v_n$ walk.

Consider the graph shown in Fig. 2.1. It has an order 5 as it contains five vertices, namely $\{A, B, C, D, E\}$. The size of the graph is 7 as it contains seven edges, namely $\{AB, AD, AE, BC, BD, BE, DE\}$.

Figure 2.2 shows a bipartite graph. Note that the two vertex sets V_1 and V_2 are disjoint. V_1 consists of the vertices $\{A, B, C\}$, and V_2 consists of the vertices $\{D, E\}$. The edges $\{AD, AE, BD, BE, CD, CE\}$ are such that each edge connects one vertex in V_1 to another vertex in V_2.

The graph in Fig. 2.3 constitutes a cycle of order 4.

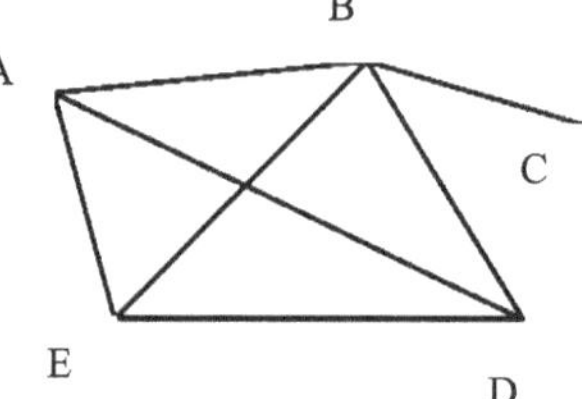

Fig. 2.1 A graph

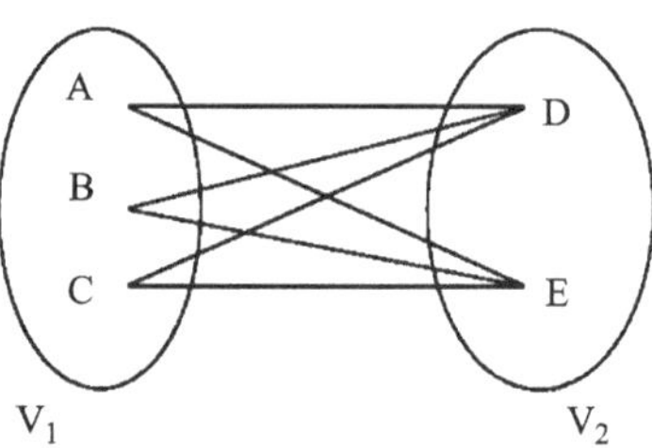

Fig. 2.2 A bipartite graph

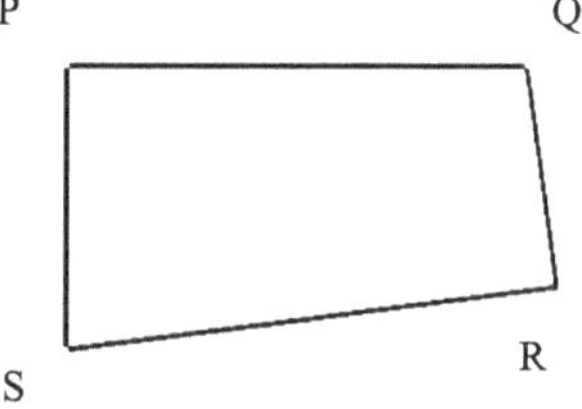

Fig. 2.3 A cycle graph

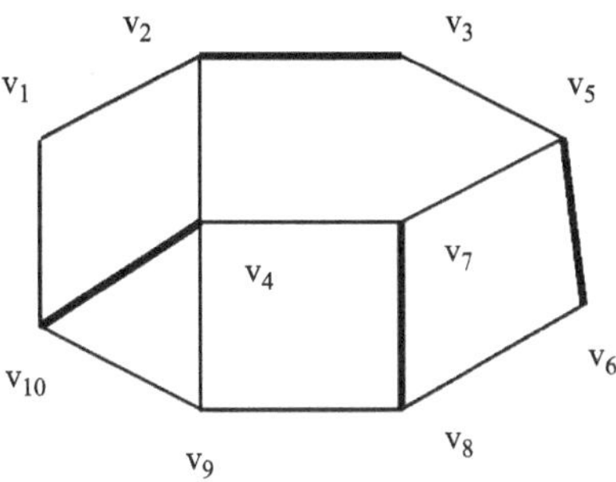

Fig. 2.4 Matching in a general graph

2.2 Matchings in Graphs

In this section, we first provide some important definitions and then present some key results on matchings in general graphs and bipartite graphs.

Definition 2.7 A *matching* M of a graph $G = (V, E)$ is a subset of the edges with the property that no two edges of M share the same node.

Definition 2.8 Edges of a graph in a matching are called *matched* edges; the other edges are called *free*. Similarly, the vertices that are not incident upon any matched edge are called *exposed*; the remaining vertices are called *free*.

Definition 2.9 A path $P = (v_1, v_2, \ldots, v_k)$ is called *alternating* if:

edges $\{v_1, v_2\}, \{v_3, v_4\}, \ldots, \{v_{2j-1}, v_{2j}\}, \ldots$ are free,
whereas edges $\{v_2, v_3\}, \{v_4, v_5\}, \ldots, \{v_{2j}, v_{2j+1}\}, \ldots$ are matched.

Definition 2.10 An alternating path $p = (v_1, v_2, \ldots, v_k)$ is called *augmenting* if both v_1 and v_k are exposed vertices.

Example 2.1 Consider Fig. 2.4 which shows a matching M in a graph G with vertices $\{v_1, \ldots, v_{10}\}$. We can then write the following:

Matched edges: $\{v_2, v_3\}, \{v_4, v_{10}\}, \{v_5, v_6\}, \{v_7, v_8\}$.
Free edges: $\{v_1, v_2\}, \{v_1, v_{10}\}, \{v_2, v_4\}, \{v_3, v_5\}, \{v_4, v_7\}, \{v_4, v_9\}, \{v_5, v_7\}, \{v_6, v_8\}, \{v_8, v_9\}, \{v_9, v_{10}\}$.
Exposed vertices: $\{v_1, v_9\}$.
An alternating path: (v_9, v_8, v_7, v_5).
An augmenting path: $(v_9, v_8, v_7, v_4, v_{10}, v_1)$.

Definition 2.11 If the edge weights of a graph are all unity, the matching problem is essentially a *Cardinality Matching* problem. A *Maximum Cardinality Matching* is a matching with a maximum number of edges.

Definition 2.12 When the cardinality of a matching is $\lfloor |V|/2 \rfloor$, the largest possible in a graph with $|V|$ nodes, we say that the matching is *complete* or *perfect*.

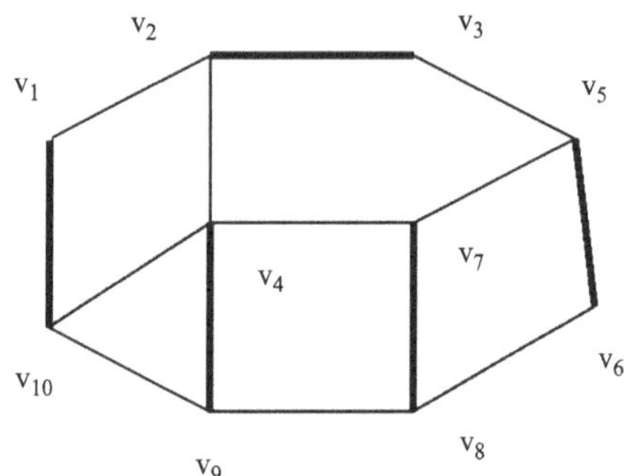

Fig. 2.5 Maximum cardinality matching in a general graph

Example 2.2 Consider Fig. 2.5 which shows a maximum cardinality matching M^* in a graph G with vertices $\{v_1, \ldots, v_{10}\}$.

Matched edges: $\{v_1, v_{10}\}, \{v_2, v_3\}, \{v_4, v_9\}, \{v_5, v_6\}, \{v_7, v_8\}$.

Since the number of vertices is 10 and the cardinality of the matching is 5, this is also an example of complete or perfect matching. Note that there are no exposed vertices and hence no augmenting paths in this figure (as opposed to Fig. 2.4).

Definition 2.13 If the edge weights are given by a function $w : E \rightarrow \Re_+$, the weight of a matching is defined as $w(M) = \sum_{e \in M} w(e)$. The *Maximum Weight Matching* problem is to determine a matching M in G that has maximum weight.

Next, we present three theorems on matchings in bipartite and general graphs. The first theorem discusses the condition for the existence of maximum matching. The next two theorems give the results for the worst-case time-complexity of two graph matching algorithms, namely, the Maximum Cardinality Minimum Weight (MCMW) matching for a bipartite graph and Maximum Weight Graph Matching (MWGM) for a general graph.

Theorem 2.1 *A matching M in a graph G is maximum if and only if there is no augmenting path in G with respect to M.*

Theorem 2.2 *The worst-case time complexity of the Maximum Cardinality Minimum Weight (MCMW) matching algorithm for a bipartite graph $G = (V_1 \cup V_2, E)$ with $|V_1| = |V_2| = n$ is $O(n^3)$.*

Theorem 2.3 *The worst-case time complexity of the Maximum Weight Graph Matching (MWGM) algorithm for a general graph $G = (V, E)$ with $|V| = n$ is $O(n^4)$.*

For detailed proofs of the above theorems and details of the matching algorithms, the interested reader can refer to [31, 33].

2.3 Isomorphism and Automorphism of Graphs

We discuss the isomorphism and automorphism of graphs with some examples. Some important results on the time complexity of the graph isomorphism problem and graph automorphism problem are also stated.

Definition 2.14 Two graphs $G_1 = (V_1, E_1)$ and $G_2 = (V_2, E_2)$ are isomorphic, denoted by $G_1 \cong G_2$, if there exists a bijection $M \subseteq V_1 \times V_2$ such that, for every pair of vertices $v_i, v_j \in V_1$ and $w_i, w_j \in V_2$ with $(v_i, w_i) \in M$ and $(v_j, w_j) \in M$, $(v_i, v_j) \in E_1$ if and only if $(w_i, w_j) \in E_2$. In such a case, M is a *graph isomorphism* from G_1 to G_2.

Definition 2.15 An *automorphism* of a graph G is a graph isomorphism between G and itself.

The set of all automorphs of a graph forms a group under the operation of composition. This group is termed the *automorphism group* of the graph. It is a well-known fact that the graph isomorphism problem (i.e., determining whether or not two graphs are isomorphic) $\in NP$. However, it can be solved in *polynomial time* for many special graphs [34]. Now, we state and prove a result on graph automorphisms for cycle graphs.

Theorem 2.4 *The automorphism group of a cycle graph C_n on $n \geq 3$ vertices is a group of order $2n$.*

Proof A cycle graph C_n on $n \geq 3$ vertices is left fixed by exactly n rotations as well as by exactly n reflections. Thus, the resulting automorphism group has order $2n$. □

Example 2.3 The two graphs G_1 and G_2 in Fig. 2.6 are isomorphic. The mapping from G_1 to G_2 is given by the following bijection:

$$M = \{(A, 1), (B, 2), (C, 3), (D, 4)\}.$$

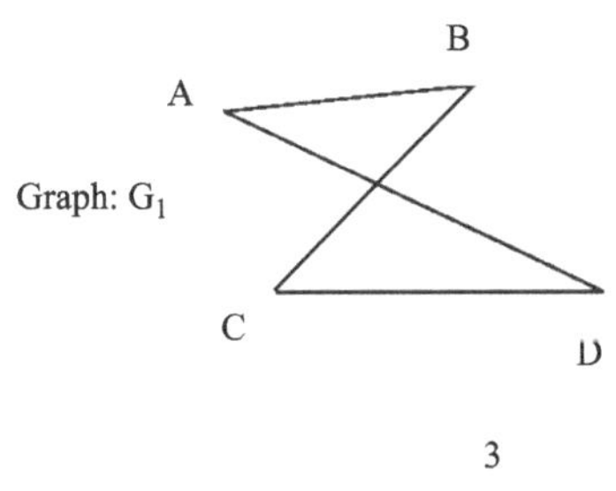

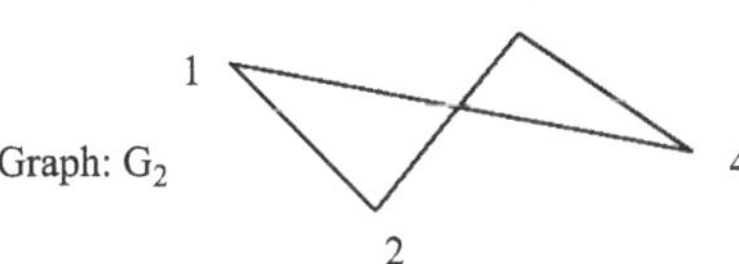

Fig. 2.6 A pair of isomorphic graphs

Example 2.4 Let C_4 be a cycle graph of order 4 with vertices $[P, Q, R, S]$, as shown in Fig. 2.3. Then from Theorem 2.4 we conclude that there exist 4 rotational automorphs and 4 reflectional automorphs, i.e., a total of 8 automorphs of C_4. The members of the automorphism group of C_4 are given by:

1. $\{P, Q, R, S\}, \{S, P, Q, R\}, \{R, S, P, Q\}, \{Q, R, S, P\}$ (these are the 4 rotational automorphs)
2. $\{Q, P, S, R\}$, $\{P, S, R, Q\}$, $\{S, R, Q, P\}$, $\{R, Q, P, S\}$ (these are the 4 reflectional automorphs)

2.4 Network Flows

In this section, we describe the basic concepts underlying network flows following [35]. As in previous sections, we state the definitions, provide some illustrative examples, and state key theorems without proofs. For the proofs of the theorems in this section, the interested reader is referred to well-known textbooks such as [35] and [36]. We end the section with a description of the Ford–Fulkerson algorithm for computing the maximum flow in a flow network.

Definition 2.16 A *flow network* $G = (V, E)$ is a directed graph in which each edge $(u, v) \in E$ has a nonnegative capacity $c(u, v) \geq 0$. Two vertices in the flow network are distinguished as a source vertex s and a sink vertex t.

Definition 2.17 A *flow* in G is a real-valued function $f : V \times V \rightarrow \Re^+$ that satisfies the following properties:

$$\forall u, v \in V, \quad f(u, v) \leq c(u, v); \tag{2.1}$$

$$\forall u, v \in V, \quad f(u, v) = -f(v, u); \tag{2.2}$$

$$\forall u \in V - \{s, t\}, \quad \sum_{v \in V} f(u, v) = 0. \tag{2.3}$$

The quantity $f(u, v)$ is called the flow from the vertex u to vertex v.

Definition 2.18 The *value* of a flow is defined as

$$|f| = \sum_{v \in V} f(s, v), \tag{2.4}$$

that is, the total flow out of the source.

Definition 2.19 Given a flow network $G = (V, E)$ and a flow f, the *residual graph* of G induced by f is $G_f = (V, E_f)$ where $E_f = \{(u, v) \in V \times V \mid c_f(u, v) > 0\}$. Here, $c_f(u, v)$ denotes the *residual capacity* of (u, v). Let $f(u, v)$ and $c(u, v)$ respectively denote the flow and capacity between u and v. Then, we can write

$$c_f(u, v) = c(u, v) - f(u, v). \tag{2.5}$$

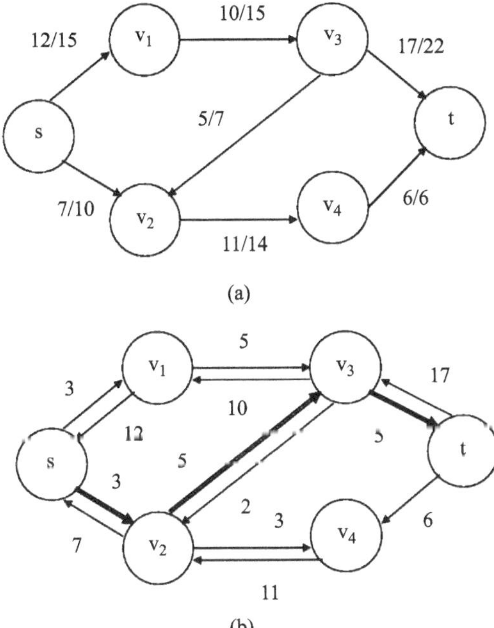

Fig. 2.7 Flow in a graph. (**a**) Flow network, (**b**) Corresponding residual network

Definition 2.20 Given a flow network $G = (V, E)$ and a flow f, an *augmenting path* p is a simple path from s to t in the residual network G_f.

Definition 2.21 We have previously defined the residual capacity for an edge in a flow network. Now, we define the residual capacity $c_f(p)$ of an augmenting path p as follows:

$$c_f(p) = \min\{c_f(u, v) \mid (u, v) \text{ is on } p\}. \tag{2.6}$$

Thus, $c_f(p)$ is the maximum amount by which a flow can be increased on each edge in the augmenting path p.

Definition 2.22 A *cut* (S, T) of a flow network $G = (V, E)$ is a partition of V into S and $T = V - S$ such that $s \in S$ and $t \in T$.

Definition 2.23 The *capacity* of a cut (S, T) is the sum of the capacities of the edges from S to T.

Example 2.5 Consider the flow network in Fig. 2.7(a). Each edge in thc flow network is labeled with a flow and a capacity. The residual network is shown in Fig. 2.7(b) with an augmenting path $p = (s, v_2, v_3, t)$. Then, using (2.5) and (2.6), we can write:

$$c_f(s, v_2) = c(s, v_2) - f(s, v_2) = 10 - 7 = 3,$$
$$c_f(v_2, v_3) = c(v_2, v_3) - f(v_2, v_3) = 7 - 5 = 2,$$

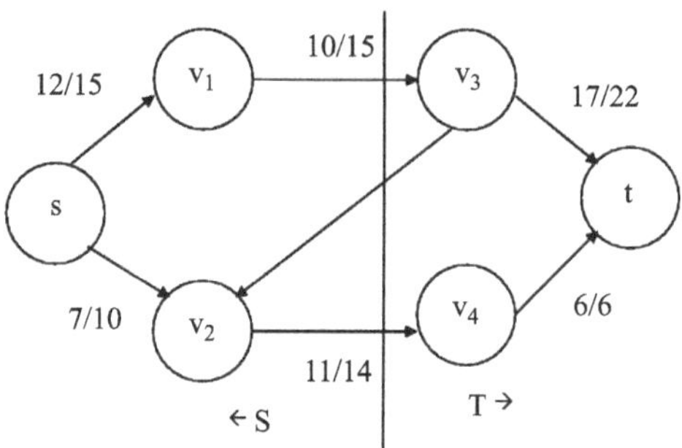

Fig. 2.8 Cut in a graph

$$c_f(v_3, t) = c(v_3, t) - f(v_3, t) = 22 - 17 = 5,$$
$$c_f(p) = \min\{c_f(s, v_2), c_f(v_2, v_3), c_f(s, v_2)\} = \min\{3, 2, 5\} = 2.$$

Example 2.6 Figure 2.8 depicts the existence of a cut in the same flow network. We can infer following from Fig. 2.8:

A cut (S, T) can be observed in the above flow network where $S = \{s, v_1, v_2\}$, $T = \{v_3, v_4, t\}$.

Capacity of this cut $= c(v_1, v_3) + c(v_2, v_4) = 15 + 14 = 29$.

Note that only edges going from S to T but not the edges in the reverse direction contribute to the capacity of a cut. Hence, only $c_f(v_1, v_3)$ and $c_f(v_2, v_4)$ are considered, and $c_f(v_3, v_2)$ is excluded when computing the capacity of the cut (S, T).

Next, we state some important theorems for flow networks. The first theorem relates the maximum flow and minimum cut in a flow network. The second theorem discusses the nature of capacity functions and the corresponding flow. Once the above definitions are extended to a multisource, multisink flow network, the third theorem establishes the equivalence of a multisource, multisink network flow problem with a single-source single-sink network flow problem.

Theorem 2.5 *For any graph, the maximum flow value from s to t is equal to the minimal cut capacity of all cuts separating s and t. This is known as Max-flow Min-Cut Theorem.*

Theorem 2.6 *If the capacity function c is integer valued, there exists a maximal flow f that is also integer valued. This is called the Integrity Theorem.*

Theorem 2.7 *Maximum flow in a graph with multiple sources $s_1, s_2, \dots, s_n$ and multiple sinks $t_1, t_2, \dots, t_n$ is induced by a maximum flow in a simple equivalent graph with an added hypersource s^* and a hypersink t^* with capacities $c(s^*, s_i) = \infty$ and $c(t_i, t^*) = \infty$. This is called the Multisource Multisink Maximum-flow Minimum-cut Theorem.*

The Ford–Fulkerson algorithm is used to find the maximum-flow in a flow network. This algorithm is based on the concepts of a residual graph, augmenting path and cut. Next, we present the basic structure of this algorithm following [35]:

Algorithm 2.1 (Ford–Fulkerson)
Input: A flow network $G(V, E)$ with source s and sink t
Output: A maximum flow f

for each edge in the flow network G
  initialize flow $f := 0$
while there exists an augmenting path p
  do augment flow f along p by adding the residual capacity
  on the augmenting path $c_f(p)$
return f

The time complexity of the Ford–Fulkerson algorithm is $O(E|f^*|)$, where f^* is the maximum flow. Note that the flow value can be increased by at least unity in each iteration of the while loop in the above algorithm, i.e., the loop can be executed at most $|f^*|$ times. The running time of the algorithm increases substantially if $|f^*|$ is quite large. For practical purposes, we often use the Edmonds–Karp algorithm for computation of the augmenting paths. A breadth-first search is employed in such cases where an augmenting path is detected as a shortest path from the source to sink. It can be shown that the Edmonds–Karp algorithm has a time complexity of $O(VE^2)$.

Chapter 3
A Statistical Primer

The aim of this chapter is to familiarize a general reader with some important statistical techniques that are used in subsequent chapters. The chapter contains four distinct sections. The first section deals with the basic concepts of probability and random variables. The second section is devoted to statistical inference which explains concepts such as the sampling distribution, point estimator, and confidence interval. The third section discusses Bayesian statistics, beginning with Bayes' theorem and concluding with Bayesian inference. The last section serves as an introduction to random fields, image restoration within a Bayesian paradigm, and some associated techniques such as stochastic relaxation. As in the previous chapter, we state the important definitions, provide illustrative examples, and mention the important results, mostly without proofs.

3.1 Probability

This section discusses some of the basic concepts of probability following the outline in [37]. Any process of observation or measurement in statistics is commonly referred to as an *experiment*.

Definition 3.1 The set of all possible outcomes of an experiment is called the *sample space*. If a sample space contains a finite or infinite (though countable) number of elements, it is called a *discrete* sample space. On the other hand, if a sample space consists of a continuum, it is called a *continuous* sample space.

Example 3.1 The sample space of an experiment consisting of rolling a pair of dice is $S = \{(x, y) \mid x = 1, 2, \dots, 6; y = 1, 2, \dots, 6\}$, where x and y respectively represent the number turned up by the first and second dice. This is an example of a discrete sample space. On the other hand, all the points on a line constitute a continuous sample space.

Definition 3.2 An *event* is a subset of a sample space.

A.S. Chowdhury, S.M. Bhandarkar, *Computer Vision-Guided Virtual Craniofacial Surgery*, Advances in Computer Vision and Pattern Recognition,
DOI 10.1007/978-0-85729-296-4_3,

Example 3.2 Let A be an event comprising of getting a sum of 8 from the rolling of two dice in the above example. Then, we can write $A = \{(2,6),(3,5),(4,4),(5,3),(6,2)\}$.

Definition 3.3 Probabilities are values of a set function, otherwise known as a *probability measure*. This function assigns real numbers to the various subsets of a sample space S. The probability of an event A is denoted as $\Pr(A)$. If an experiment results in any one of N distinct though equally likely outcomes and if n of these outcomes considered together constitute an event A, then the probability of the event A is

$$\Pr(A) = n/N. \tag{3.1}$$

Example 3.3 Consider the preceding example of rolling of a pair of dice. Let us find the probability of the event A of getting a sum of 8 from the rolling of two dice.

There are a total of $6^2 = 36$ equally likely outcomes of rolling a pair of dice. So, in this case, $N = 36$.

From Example 3.2, there are 5 different outcomes which can constitute the event A. So, in this case, $n = 5$.

Therefore, using (3.1), $\Pr(A) = 5/36$.

Definition 3.4 If A and B are any two events in a sample space S and $\Pr(A) \neq 0$, the conditional probability of B given A is

$$\Pr(B|A) = \Pr(A \cap B)/\Pr(A). \tag{3.2}$$

Example 3.4 Let us continue with the same experiment of rolling a pair of dice and find the conditional probability of getting a sum of 8 from the rolling of two dice given that one die generates an even number. In this case, the event A is that a die generates an even number, i.e., $\{2,4,6\}$.

So, $\Pr(A) = 3/6$.

If we consider two dice, we can think of $A = \{(2,1),\ldots,(2,6),(4,1),\ldots,(4,6),(6,1),\ldots,(6,6)\}$.

The event B is getting a sum of 8 from the rolling of two dice.

So, $B = \{(2,6),(3,5),(4,4),(5,3),(6,2)\}$.

Therefore, $A \cap B = \{(2,6),(4,4),(6,2)\}$ and $\Pr(A \cap B) = 3/36$.

So, $\Pr(B|A) = \frac{3/36}{3/6} = 1/6$.

Definition 3.5 If S is a sample space with a probability measure and X is a real-valued function defined over the elements of S, then X is called a *random variable*. We use an uppercase letter to express the random variable and the corresponding lowercase letter to denote the value of the random variable, e.g., $\Pr(X = x)$ represents the probability that the random variable X will assume the value x. Analogously to the definition of a sample space, if a random variable has a finite or countably infinite range, it is called a *discrete random variable*. In the case where the range is a continuum, the random variable is called a *continuous random variable*.

Example 3.5 With reference to the previous example, the random variable X (denoting the sum of the numbers returned by the dice) is a discrete random variable as it takes on the value 8 on a finite range $\{(2,6),(3,5),(4,4),(5,3),(6,2)\}$.

Definition 3.6 If X is a discrete random variable, the function given by $f(x) = \Pr(X = x)$ for each x within the range of X is called the *probability distribution* of X. Examples of common probability distributions include the *Binomial distribution* and the *Geometric distribution*. In the case of discrete random variables, the probability distributions are also known as probability mass functions.

The Binomial distribution essentially gives the probability of obtaining x successful outcomes in n trials. Let θ be the probability of a successful outcome. A random variable X has a binomial distribution if its probability distribution is given by

$$b(x; n, \theta) = \binom{n}{x} \theta^x (1-\theta)^{(n-x)}. \tag{3.3}$$

Definition 3.7 A function with values $f(x)$, defined over the set of all real numbers, is called the *probability distribution function* of the continuous random variable X iff

$$\Pr(a \leq X \leq b) = \int_a^b f(x)\,dx. \tag{3.4}$$

For continuous random variables, the probability distributions are also known as probability density functions.

A continuous random variable X, taking all real values in the range $(-\infty, \infty)$ is said to follow a normal distribution with parameters μ and σ iff it has the following probability density function:

$$n(x; \mu, \sigma) = \frac{1}{\sigma\sqrt{2\pi}} \exp\left(-\frac{(x-\mu)^2}{2\sigma^2}\right). \tag{3.5}$$

Definition 3.8 If X is a discrete random variable and $f(x)$ is the value of the probability distribution at $X = x$, the *expectation* of X is given by

$$E(X) = \sum_x x f(x). \tag{3.6}$$

For a continuous random variable X with probability density $f(x)$ at $X = x$, the *expectation* of X is given by

$$E(X) = \int_{-\infty}^{\infty} x f(x)\,dx. \tag{3.7}$$

The expectation is also known as the *mean* of the distribution of X and is denoted by μ.

Definition 3.9 If X is a discrete random variable and $f(x)$ is the value of the probability distribution at $X = x$, the *variance* of X is given by

$$\mathrm{Var}(X) = \sum_{x} (x - \mu)^2 f(x). \tag{3.8}$$

For a continuous random variable X with probability density $f(x)$ at $X = x$, the *variance* of X is given by

$$\mathrm{Var}(X) = \int_{-\infty}^{\infty} (x - \mu)^2 f(x)\, dx. \tag{3.9}$$

The variance of the distribution of X is denoted by σ^2. The standard deviation of the distribution is given by the square root of the variance, i.e., $\mathrm{sd}(X) = \sigma$.

Definition 3.10 If X is a discrete random variable and $f(x)$ is the value of the probability distribution at $X = x$, the *mode* of X is that value of x for which $f(x)$ occurs maximum number of times. For a continuous random variable X with probability density $f(x)$ at $X = x$, the *mode* of X is that value of x for which $f(x)$ attains a maximum.

3.2 Statistical Inference

This section discusses some preliminary yet fundamental concepts underlying statistical inference such as random samples, sampling distributions, Central Limit Theorem, point estimation of a parameter, and estimation by confidence intervals. For further details on any of the concepts dealt with in this section, we refer the interested reader to [38].

Definition 3.11 A *population* is the complete set of possible measurements for which inferences are to be made. On the other hand, a *sample* is the set of measurements, actually collected from a statistical population, in the course of an investigation.

Definition 3.12 A *random sample* of size n from a population $f(x)$ is a collection of n independent random variables $X_1, X_2, \ldots, X_n$, each having the distribution $f(x)$.

The distribution described by $f(x)$ can be either discrete or continuous. The probabilistic condition of independence is inherent in the definition of the random samples. It is important to note that in a process of random sampling, the same set of random variables prior to observation becomes a set of numbers after the observation.

Definition 3.13 A *statistic* is a function of the sample observations.

A statistic is essentially a sample measure. Typical sample measures include, among others, the sample mean and sample variance.

Definition 3.14 The probability distribution of a statistic, which is itself a random variable, is called the *sampling distribution* of the statistic.

Let us consider a random sample of size n. Let $\bar{X}$ be the sample mean, μ be the population mean, and σ^2 be the population variance. Then, the following results can be easily shown:

$$\begin{aligned} E(\bar{X}) &= \mu, \\ \text{Var}(\bar{X}) &= \frac{\sigma^2}{n}, \\ \text{sd}(\bar{X}) &= \frac{\sigma^2}{\sqrt{n}}. \end{aligned} \tag{3.10}$$

Now, we state two important results about the sampling distribution of the sample mean $\bar{X}$ of a normal and arbitrary population. In the case of a random sampling from a population that follows a normal distribution with mean μ and standard deviation σ,

$$\bar{X} \sim \mathcal{N}\left(\mu, \frac{\sigma}{\sqrt{n}}\right). \tag{3.11}$$

Theorem 3.1 *The* Central Limit Theorem *states that the distribution of $\bar{X}$ in case of an arbitrary population of size n with mean μ and standard deviation σ follows an approximate normal distribution with mean μ and standard deviation $\frac{\sigma}{\sqrt{n}}$ in case of a large n. So, we can write*

$$Z = \frac{\bar{X} - \mu}{(\sigma/\sqrt{n})} \sim \mathcal{N}(0, 1). \tag{3.12}$$

With the above background, we now introduce very basic concepts about *statistical inference*. Statistical inference can be considered as a generalization about the population parameters from an analysis of the sample data. As mentioned in the beginning of this section, we limit our discussion to point estimation of a parameter and estimation by confidence intervals.

In order to estimate the unknown value of a parameter θ, a *point estimator* $\hat{\theta}$ is designed. The point estimator, more commonly referred to as an estimator, is a function of the sample observations. An estimator $\hat{\theta}$ is called *unbiased* for a parameter θ if $E(\hat{\theta}) = \theta$, whatever the true value of θ. The property of unbiasedness precludes the systematic overestimation or underestimation of the parameter θ in the case of repeated samplings. The accuracy of estimation depends on the standard deviation of the sampling distribution of the estimator. For this purpose, the *minimum variance unbiased estimator* of θ can be selected. The standard deviation of the estimator $\hat{\theta}$ is called its *standard error* and is denoted by $S.E.(\hat{\theta})$.

Note that a point estimator only provides a single number as an estimate of the parameter. An alternative technique, called the *confidence interval estimation*, produces an interval of values that is likely to contain the true value of the parameter. Let $(1-\alpha)$ be a specified high probability value, and L and U be functions of a random sample $X_1, X_2, \ldots, X_n$ such that

$$\Pr[L < \theta < U] = 1 - \alpha. \tag{3.13}$$

The interval (L, U) is called a $100(1-\alpha)\%$ confidence interval for the parameter, and $(1-\alpha)$ is called the confidence level associated with the interval. From the Central Limit Theorem, the sample mean $\bar{X} \sim \mathcal{N}(\mu, \frac{\sigma}{\sqrt{n}})$. It is a fact that the probability that a normal random variable will lie within 1.96 standard deviations of its mean is 0.95. So, by letting $\theta = \bar{X}$, $L = \mu - 1.96\frac{\sigma}{\sqrt{n}}$, $U = \mu + 1.96\frac{\sigma}{\sqrt{n}}$, and $(1-\alpha) = 0.95$ in (3.13), we can write

$$\Pr\left[\mu - 1.96\frac{\sigma}{\sqrt{n}} < \bar{X} < \mu + 1.96\frac{\sigma}{\sqrt{n}}\right] = 0.95. \tag{3.14}$$

We can rewrite (3.14) as follows:

$$\Pr\left[\bar{X} - 1.96\frac{\sigma}{\sqrt{n}} < \mu < \bar{X} + 1.96\frac{\sigma}{\sqrt{n}}\right] = 0.95. \tag{3.15}$$

Finally, the more generalized version of (3.15) for a $100(1-\alpha)\%$ confidence interval for μ can be written as

$$\Pr\left[\bar{X} - z_{\alpha/2}\frac{\sigma}{\sqrt{n}} < \mu < \bar{X} + z_{\alpha/2}\frac{\sigma}{\sqrt{n}}\right] = (1-\alpha). \tag{3.16}$$

Example 3.6 Given a random sample of 256 observations from a population for which μ is unknown and $\sigma = 8$. The sample mean is found to be 40.8. Provide a 95% confidence interval for μ.

We have the sample size $n = 256$, which is large. So, from the Central Limit Theorem, the normal approximation to the distribution of $\bar{X}$ is valid. Thus, we simply use (3.15) to solve this problem. The 95% confidence interval for μ is obtained as $(40.8 - 1.96\frac{8}{\sqrt{256}}, 40.8 + 1.96\frac{8}{\sqrt{256}}) = (39.82, 41.78)$.

3.3 Bayesian Statistics

In this section, we focus on some basic aspects of Bayesian statistics. This section develops upon some of the concepts presented in the previous two sections. We begin with Bayes' theorem and provide an illustrative example. Next, we discuss prior, likelihood, and posterior distributions in the context of Bayesian inference in a more general manner. The material presented in this section follows well-known textbooks on Bayesian statistics such as [37] and [39].

Theorem 3.2 Bayes' theorem *states that:*

If the events $B_1, B_2, \ldots, B_k$ *constitute a partition of the sample space* S *and* $\Pr(B_i) \neq 0$ *for* $i = 1, 2, \ldots, k$, *then for any event* $A \in S$ *such that* $\Pr(A) \neq 0$,

$$\Pr(B_m|A) = \frac{\Pr(B_m)\Pr(A|B_m)}{\sum_{i=1}^{k}\Pr(B_i)\cdot\Pr(A|B_i)} \tag{3.17}$$

for $m = 1, 2, \ldots, k$.

Example 3.7 In a certain community, 8 percent of all adults over 50 have diabetes. If a health service in this community correctly diagnoses 95 percent of all persons with diabetes as having the disease and incorrectly diagnoses 2 percent of all persons without diabetes as having the disease, find the probability that a person over 50 diagnosed by the health service as having diabetes actually has the disease.

Let us first identify the events associated with this problem.

A is the event of a person over 50 diagnosed by the health service.

B_1 is the event that an adult over 50 actually has the diabetes. So, $\Pr(B_1) = 0.08$.

B_2 is the event that an adult over 50 does not have the diabetes.

So, $\Pr(B_2) = 1 - \Pr(B_1) = 0.92$.

From the available information, $\Pr(A|B_1) = 0.95$ and $\Pr(A|B_2) = 0.02$.

We need to find $\Pr(B_1|A)$. Following (3.10), we can write $\Pr(B_1|A) = \frac{\Pr(B_1)\Pr(A|B_1)}{\Pr(B_1)\Pr(A|B_1)+\Pr(B_2)\Pr(A|B_2)}$.

Substituting all the relevant values, we get $\Pr(B_1|A) = \frac{(0.08)(0.95)}{(0.08)(0.95)+(0.92)(0.02)} = 0.8051$.

Bayesian statistical conclusions can be made about a parameter θ, or an unobserved data $\tilde{y}$ on the basis of probability statements. The probability statements are conditional on the observed value of y. Bayes' theorem provides the formulation for making probability statements about θ given y as follows:

$$\Pr(\theta|y) = \frac{\Pr(\theta)\Pr(y|\theta)}{\Pr(y)}. \tag{3.18}$$

In the discrete case, $\Pr(y) = \sum_\theta \Pr(\theta)\Pr(y|\theta)$. In the continuous case, $\Pr(y) = \int \Pr(\theta)\Pr(y|\theta)\,d\theta$. In (3.18), $\Pr(\theta)$ is called the *prior* distribution, $\Pr(y|\theta)$ is called the *likelihood* function, and $\Pr(\theta|y)$ is known as the *posterior* distribution.

After the data y from a process have been observed, we can predict an unknown observable, $\tilde{y}$, from the same process. The distribution of $\tilde{y}$ is called the *posterior predictive* distribution. The distribution of $\tilde{y}$ is *posterior* in nature because it is conditional on the observed y. On the other hand, the distribution of $\tilde{y}$ is also predictive because it is a prediction for an observable $\tilde{y}$. We can write

$$\Pr(\tilde{y}|y) = \int \Pr(\tilde{y}|\theta)\Pr(\theta|y)\,d\theta. \tag{3.19}$$

It can be shown that the posterior predictive distribution has the same mean as the posterior distribution, whereas its variance is equal to the sum of the prior predictive variance of the model and the variance of the posterior distribution. We can further construct Bayesian prediction intervals, in a manner similar to the estimation of confidence intervals described in the previous section. The Bayesian prediction intervals are also known as *Credible Sets*.

3.4 Random Fields, Bayesian Restoration, and Stochastic Relaxation

In this section, we discuss key concepts related to random fields, Bayesian image restoration, and stochastic relaxation. We follow the treatments of the above topics given in [40, 41], and [43]:

Definition 3.15 Let $F = \{F_1, \ldots, F_m\}$ be a family of random variables defined on a set S in which each random variable F_i takes a value f_i in the set of labels L. The family F is called a *random field.*

Definition 3.16 F is said to be a *Markov Random Field* (*MRF*) on a collection of sites S with respect to a neighborhood system N if and only if the following two conditions are satisfied:

$$\begin{aligned} &\Pr(f) > 0 \quad \forall f \in L \quad \text{(positivity)}, \\ &\Pr(f_i \mid f_{S-(i)}) = \Pr(f_i \mid f_{N_i}) \quad \text{(Markovianity)}, \end{aligned} \tag{3.20}$$

where $S - (i)$ denotes the set difference, $f_{S-(i)}$ denotes the set of labels at the sites $S - (i)$, and $f_{N_i} = (f_{i'} | i' \in N_i)$ denotes the set of labels at the sites neighboring site i.

In the context of digital image processing, an image pixel can be considered as a site. For an 8-bit image, the set of quantized intensities $\{0, 1, 2, \ldots, 255\}$ can be viewed as the set of discrete labels at the pixel sites. Each pixel in a given image can assume one of the above intensities. Thus, an image can be essentially represented as an MRF. An image of size $m \times m$ corresponds to a regular lattice of size $m \times m$ which can be treated as comprising of a collection of sites S. On such a lattice, we can define various neighborhood systems N such as a first-order neighborhood system comprising of the 4-neighbors of a pixel site and a second-order neighborhood system of the 8-neighbors of a pixel site. The pair (S, N) constitutes a graph where S contains the nodes and N determines the links between the nodes according to the neighboring relationship.

Definition 3.17 A *clique* c is defined as a subset of sites S wherein each pair of distinct sites in c are neighbors. A first-order clique system c_1 is a collection of single pixel sites $c_1 = \{i \mid i \in S\}$. A second-order clique system c_2 is a collection of all pairs of neighboring pixel sites $c_2 = \{(i_1, i_2) \mid i_1, i_2 \in S \text{ are neighbors}\}$. Higher-order clique systems $c_3, c_4, \ldots$ can be similarly defined. The collection of all cliques of all possible orders for (S, N) can be written as $C = c_1 \cup c_2 \ldots$.

The positivity condition in (3.20) ensures that the joint probability $\Pr(f)$ of a random field F is uniquely determined by its local conditional probabilities. Markovianity, on the other hand, signifies that only the neighboring labels directly influence each other. An MRF is said to be *homogeneous* if $\Pr(f_i \mid f_{N_i})$ is independent of the position of i in S. The MRFs on spatial indices are exactly equivalent to Markov processes on time indices. In order to describe an MRF, one can either use joint probabilities or conditional probabilities. The joint distribution is not at all apparent, and it is extremely difficult to design appropriate functions to denote conditional probabilities based on local characteristics. This problem is solved by the application of the *Hammersley–Clifford theorem*. We first define a Gibbs Random Field (GRF) and then show the equivalence of an MRF and a GRF using the Hammersley–Clifford theorem.

Definition 3.18 A set of random variables F is said to be a *Gibbs Random Field* (*GRF*) on S with respect to N if and only if its configurations obey a Gibbs distribution. A Gibbs distribution takes the following form:

$$\Pr(f) = Z^{-1} \exp^{-U(f)/T}, \tag{3.21}$$

where the partition function Z is given by

$$Z = \sum_{f \in F} \exp^{-U(f)/T}. \tag{3.22}$$

The parameter T in (3.21) is termed as the temperature, and $U(f)$ is termed as the energy function. The energy function can be expressed in terms of the clique potentials V_c as follows:

$$U(f) = \sum_{c \in C} V_c(f). \tag{3.23}$$

The value of the clique potential $V_c(f)$ in (3.23) depends only on the local site configurations associated with clique c. As is evident, the terminology for the GRF is derived from the rich field of statistical physics where Gibbs distributions are used to model the energy states of ferromagnets, ideal gases, and binary alloys. The function V_c in such cases denotes contributions due to external fields (represented by the first-order cliques), pair interactions (represented by the second-order cliques), and so on. A GRF is *homogeneous* if $U(f)$ is independent of the relative position of the clique c in S. A GRF is said to be *isotropic* if $U(f)$ is independent of the orientation of clique c in S.

Theorem 3.3 *F is an MRF on S with respect to N if and only if F is a GRF on S with respect to N. This result is known as the* Hammersley–Clifford theorem.

For the proof of the Hammersley–Clifford theorem, the interested reader is referred to [42]. By specifying the clique potential V_c, one can specify the energy function $U(f)$ using (3.23). Consequently, using (3.21), the joint probability $\Pr(f)$ can be specified from the energy function $U(f)$. Finally, by invoking the Hammersley–Clifford theorem, the MRF can be specified by actually specifying the GRF and invoking the MRF–GRF equivalence. The properties of homogeneity and isotropy of the GRF carry over to its equivalent MRF.

Next, we explain prior and posterior distributions and Maximum A Posteriori (MAP) estimation in the context of Bayesian image restoration. Let us assume that

Π is a probability distribution defined on a set of preexisting images $\mathbf{X}$. As Π depends on the individual preexisting images $x \in \mathbf{X}$ and not on the observed data y, it is considered a *prior* distribution. Let us further assume $\Pr(y|x)$ to be the probability of observing the data y if x is the correct image. Thus, $\Pr(y|x)$ can be deemed a *likelihood* function. Following *Bayes' theorem*, we can derive the conditional probability of $x \in \mathbf{X}$ given y as follows:

$$\Pr(x|y) = \frac{\Pi(x)\Pr(y|x)}{\sum_z \Pi(z)\Pr(z|y)}. \tag{3.24}$$

Since $\Pr(.|y)$ can be looked upon as an adjustment to Π to account for the observed data y, it is considered the *posterior* distribution of x given y. A *mode* $x^*(y)$ of the posterior distribution $\Pr(.|y)$ is called a *Maximum Posterior Estimate* (*MAP*) of x given y. For Gibbsian posterior distributions, the MAP estimates are the minimizers of the posterior energy. In the context of an image restoration problem that is cast in the Bayesian paradigm, the goal is often to determine the MAP estimate from the available degraded image data, the likelihood function, and knowledge of the image intensity distribution or prior distribution. It is relevant to mention that the posterior distribution can serve as an important tool for more general image analysis and can be used for different purposes, such as parameter estimation and design of suitable statistical tests for detection of specific objects in the image, in addition to image restoration via MAP estimation. The determination of the MAP estimate poses a considerable computational challenge. Even for a small binary image of size 64×64, the number of possible intensity images or the cardinality of the set of all possible configurations is $2^{64\times 64}$, a prohibitively large number for any practical computer. For a prior distribution or energy function that is Gibbsian (which is usually the case with an image), it can be shown that the posterior distribution or energy function is also Gibbsian. This is an example of *conjugacy* since the posterior distribution follows the same parametric form as the prior distribution. As mentioned before, one needs to minimize the Gibbsian posterior distribution or energy function in order to arrive at the MAP estimate. Stochastic relaxation algorithms are often employed as the optimization technique for determining the MAP estimate.

A *stochastic relaxation algorithm* is a nondeterministic, iterative algorithm commonly employed to determine the MAP estimate. In contrast to deterministic algorithms that are typically based on variations of hill climbing search, local search, or gradient descent search, a stochastic relaxation algorithm permits both positive and negative changes to the objective function, hence potentially allowing it to escape from local minima. MAP estimation via stochastic relaxation results in the asymptotic realization of an irreducible aperiodic Markov chain with an equilibrium measure or equivalently a stationary distribution (also termed as a target distribution). A sampling algorithm generates a sequence of samples or solution configurations from the target distribution such that the distribution of the samples or solution configurations asymptotically converges to the target distribution. The *Gibbs Sampler* is one example of a stochastic relaxation algorithm, which generates new samples or solution configurations from a target Gibbs distribution. The target Gibbs distribution or random field in the present context refers to the posterior distribution or random field.

Part II
Virtual Craniofacial Reconstruction

Chapter 4
Virtual Single-Fracture Mandibular Reconstruction

4.1 Motivation

In this chapter, we discuss in detail the various aspects of the problem of virtual mandibular reconstruction in the presence of a single fracture. Much of this discussion is applicable not only to situations that involve exclusively a single fracture, but also to multiple fracture scenarios wherein the fractures are fixated one at a time in the operating room. Thus, the problem of mandibular reconstruction in the case of a single fracture assumes paramount importance in most craniofacial trauma cases.

The plastic surgeon in the operating room restores the form and function of the fractured bone elements in the craniofacial skeleton typically by first exposing all the bone fragments, then returning them to their normal configuration (a process referred to as fracture reduction), and finally maintaining these reduced bone fragments with rigid screws and plates. This approach is termed the *Open Reduction Internal Fixation* (ORIF) protocol in the surgical literature. However, there are several critical and inherent limitations to this current, standard approach. Visualizing the bone fragments in order to reduce them necessitates their exposure which consequently reduces the attached blood supply and also increases the operating time. To improve the blood supply, one can decrease the extent of dissection. However this means not being able to visualize the entire fracture, which could lead to potential misalignments of the bone fragments. In this chapter we propose and describe a scheme that could reduce significantly the exposure time and operating time without sacrificing surgical precision. Additionally, the proposed scheme would result in a substantial reduction in the operative and postoperative trauma to the patient while decreasing significantly the cost of surgery.

4.2 Chapter Organization

The remainder of the chapter is organized into ten different sections. In Sect. 4.3, we discuss the existing literature on craniofacial reconstruction along with some computer vision algorithms that can be brought to bear for this purpose and also

A.S. Chowdhury, S.M. Bhandarkar, *Computer Vision-Guided Virtual Craniofacial Surgery*, Advances in Computer Vision and Pattern Recognition,
DOI 10.1007/978-0-85729-296-4_4,

highlight our contribution. In Sect. 4.4, a series of image processing tasks such as thresholding and connected component labeling are described. This is followed by Sect. 4.5, which discusses three surface matching algorithms using type-0 constraints. The three subsections within this section, i.e., Sects. 4.5.1, 4.5.2, and 4.5.3, are respectively devoted to the descriptions of the ICP algorithm, the DARCES algorithm, and the hybrid DARCES–ICP algorithm.

In Sect. 4.6, we show how effective modeling of the existing irregularities on a fracture surface can potentially improve the matching accuracy. This section, like the previous one, also contains three subsections. In Sects. 4.6.1 and 4.6.2, we describe surface irregularity modeling approaches based on the theory of mean and Gaussian curvatures and on fuzzy set theory, respectively. Section 4.6.3 describes two reward–penalty schemes that serve to incorporate the extracted surface irregularity information within the surface matching process. Section 4.7 discusses an alternative scheme to improve the surface matching accuracy by exploitation of type-1 constraints. Sections 4.7.1, 4.7.2, and 4.7.3 respectively describe the generation of multiple initial states as cycle graph automorphs, selection of the best initial state using type-1 constraints accompanied by shape knowledge, and a hybrid Geometric-ICP algorithm for surface matching. In Sect. 4.8, we explore the bilateral symmetry of the mandible. Section 4.9 provides a detailed analysis and modeling of the biomechanical stability of the mandible. In Sect. 4.10, we combine the bilateral symmetry and biomechanical stability criteria with the previously described hybrid DARCES–ICP surface matching algorithm to enhance the performance of the virtual reconstruction procedure. In Sect. 4.11, we present experimental results and their analysis. Finally, we conclude the chapter in Sect. 4.12 and outline directions for future research.

4.3 Related Work and Our Contribution

A lot of interesting research has been conducted over the past decade in various aspects of automation of craniofacial and maxillofacial surgery. The mass tensor model has been used for fast prediction of soft tissue deformation in [21], whereas the mass-spring model has been used for fast surgical simulation from CT data in [44]. The problem of building a virtual craniofacial patient from CT data has been addressed in [20]. A reconstruction approach involving complete 3D modeling of the solid high-detailed structure of the craniofacial skeleton, starting from the information present in the 3D diagnostic CT images, can be found in [45]. A survey with detailed information about the reconstruction of anatomic models from craniofacial image data can be found in [46]. The Iterative Closest Point (ICP) [47] algorithm is seen to be a popular computer vision algorithm for surface registration in the field of medical imaging [48]. Variants of the ICP algorithm in the context of medical imaging that incorporate certain statistical concepts such as Expectation Maximization (EM) can be found in [49]. A desirable property of the ICP algorithm is that it yields an accurate registration given a good initial solution. An alternative surface registration algorithm, called the Data Aligned Rigidity Constrained Exhaustive Search (DARCES) algorithm, which incorporates a Random Sample Consensus

(RANSAC) model fitting approach [50], is also popular in the context of medical imaging because of its robustness to outliers [51]. A two-stage general framework based on block matching strategies, for the purpose of robust rigid medical image registration, has been proposed in [52].

The first contribution of this chapter lies in solving the 3D correspondence problem using the Maximum Cardinality Minimum Weight (MCMW) Bipartite Graph Matching algorithm. The second contribution is the formulation of the hybrid DARCES–ICP algorithm [53]. The synergism between the ICP and DARCES algorithms is exploited in three different ways [54]. The synergetic combination of the two algorithms, where the output of the DARCES algorithm is fed as input to the ICP algorithm, is observed to result in an improved surface matching algorithm with a considerable reduction in both, the mean squared error (MSE) and the execution time. The third contribution of the work lies in the modeling the irregularities of the fracture surfaces using the theory of mean and Gaussian curvatures and the theory of fuzzy sets [55]. The fourth contribution lies in the generation of multiple initial solutions for the ICP algorithm using concepts from graph automorphism and the resulting formulation of the hybrid Geometric-ICP algorithm [56, 57].

The last, but not the least, contribution is the incorporation of bilateral symmetry and biomechanical stability of the human mandible in the virtual reconstruction process. The anatomy of the human mandible clearly exhibits bilateral symmetry. Furthermore, basic biomechanical principles postulate that the most stable state for a solid body is the state with minimum energy and that this fact should be applicable to the human mandible as well. Since both the ICP and DARCES algorithms, in their original formulation, are essentially data driven and purely local in nature, they cannot, in their original formulation, explicitly guarantee the preservation of either the global shape symmetry or the biomechanical stability of the reconstructed human mandible. The incorporation of anatomical shape knowledge in medical image registration has been discussed in [58, 59]. However, we go one step further in our reconstruction paradigm. A composite reconstruction metric is introduced and expressed as a linear combination of three different terms, namely (a) the mean squared surface matching error (MSE), (b) a global shape symmetry term, and (c) a surface area term which is shown to be a measure of biomechanical stability. An angular perturbation scheme is used to optimize the composite reconstruction metric. Thus, we explore and address, in an innovative manner, the preservation of the anatomical shape and the biomechanical stability of the reconstructed mandible in the virtual domain (which may not always be possible in the operating room). As shown in this chapter, this composite reconstruction scheme integrates computer vision algorithms with concepts from biomechanics and graph theory to yield a more accurate reconstruction [60].

4.4 Image Processing

The input to the computer vision-guided virtual craniofacial reconstruction system is a sequence of 2D grayscale images of a fractured human mandible, generated

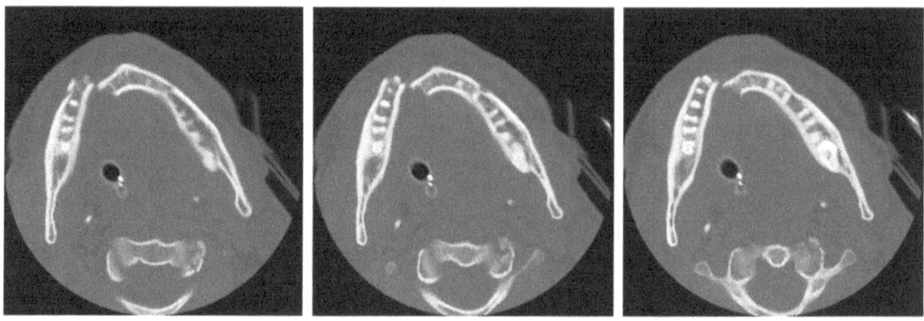

Fig. 4.1 A real patient CT image sequence of a fractured mandible. The images in (**a**), (**b**), and (**c**) are three consecutive slices in the CT image sequence

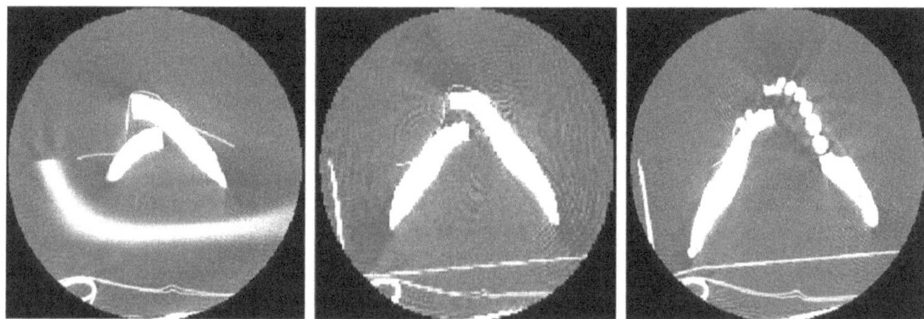

Fig. 4.2 A CT image sequence of a fractured phantom mandible. The image in (**a**) is a slice appearing at the *beginning* of the sequence, the image in (**b**) is a slice appearing in the *middle* of the sequence, and the image in (**c**) is a slice appearing at the *end* of the sequence. These slices are not consecutive

using Computed Tomography (CT). Figure (4.1) shows a CT image sequence obtained from a real (human) patient where the images shown in Figs. 4.1(a), (b), and (c) represent three consecutive CT slices. Figure 4.2 shows three nonconsecutive CT image slices of a fractured phantom mandible, where the slice shown in Fig. 4.2(a) occurs at the beginning of the CT image sequence, the slice shown in Fig. 4.2(b) occurs in the middle of the CT image sequence, and the slice shown in Fig. 4.2(c) occurs at the end of the CT image sequence. A series of image processing tasks are undertaken before using the various surface matching algorithms to register the two fractured bone fragments. The results of the image processing operations on the real (human) patient CT data in Fig. 4.1 are shown in Fig. 4.3 and on the phantom CT data in Fig. 4.2 are shown in Fig. 4.4. The software resulting from the implementation of the surface matching algorithms and image processing tasks is currently integrated into a JAVA-based package for computer-assisted reconstructive plastic surgery called *InSilicoSurgeon* (©The University of Georgia Research Foundation Inc., 2004). A brief description of the image processing tasks is given below:

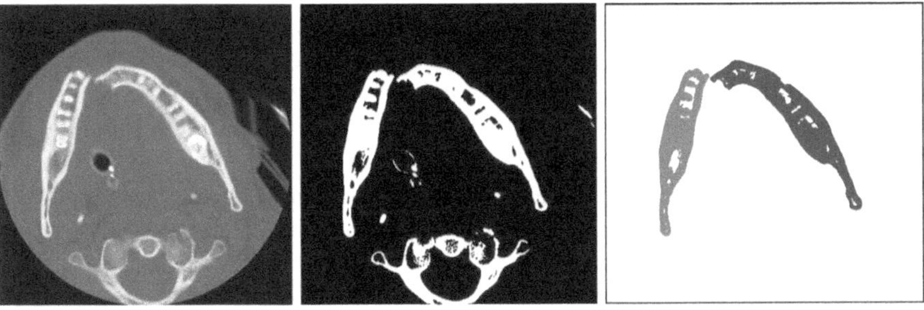

Fig. 4.3 (**a**) A typical 2D CT slice from a real patient CT sequence. (**b**) The CT slice after entropy-based thresholding. (**c**) The CT slice after connected component labeling and size filtering. In (**c**), the two fractured mandibular fragments are represented by two different intensity values

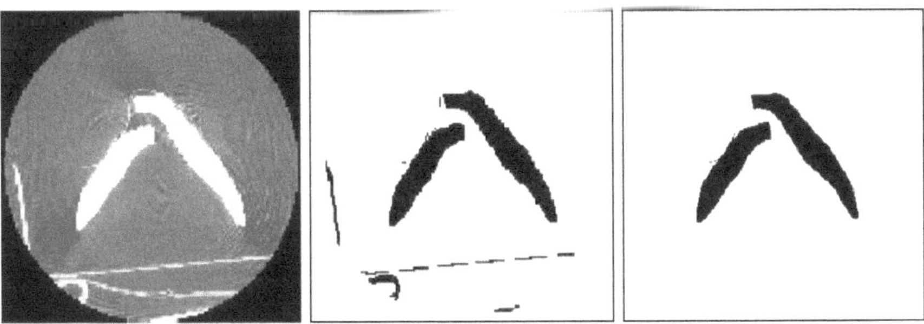

Fig. 4.4 (**a**) A typical 2D CT slice from a phantom CT sequence. (**b**) The CT slice after simple thresholding. (**c**) The CT slice after connected component labeling and size filtering. In (**b**) and (**c**), the grayscale value 0 (i.e., *color black*) is used to represent the mandibular bone fragments and artifacts

4.4.1 Thresholding

Two types of thresholding algorithms were used in *InSilicoSurgeon*©. For the phantom CT images, the bright components (with higher Hounsfield unit values [61]) represent the fractured mandible (bone) fragments, whereas the dark areas (with relatively lower Hounsfield unit values) represent soft tissue. Hence, the threshold value for the binarization of the CT image was not difficult to select, and simple thresholding was observed to be sufficient. Based on a priori knowledge, a pixel with grayscale value above a certain threshold value T was classified as belonging to the object of interest and represented using the grayscale value 0 (i.e., the color black) as shown in Fig. 4.4(b). Thus, for a grayscale CT image slice $G(i, j)$, we obtain a binary image $B(i, j)$ given by

$$B(i, j) = \begin{cases} 0 & \text{if } G(i, j) > T, \\ 1 & \text{otherwise.} \end{cases} \tag{4.1}$$

However, for real (human) patient CT data, the selection of the appropriate threshold is not obvious since the CT images typically contain objects or artifacts of different intensities (varying Hounsfield unit values). For example, a fractured mandibular fragment could contain cavities, dental fillings, crowns, and other dental prostheses. In such cases, entropy-based thresholding [62] was found to perform better than simple thresholding. In the case of entropy-based thresholding, the threshold value (represented by the variable T in (1)) is determined via maximization of the interclass entropy computed from the grayscale histogram of the CT image. The entropy, in general, is a probabilistic measure of the uncertainty of an event. For an image, the entropy S_c for each grayscale class c (consisting of several grayscale values) can be computed using the grayscale histogram as follows:

$$S_c = -\sum_{k \in G_c} p(k) \log_2\bigl(p(k)\bigr), \tag{4.2}$$

where $p(k)$ is the probability of a pixel having a grayscale value k, and G_c is the set of grayscale values for class c. In the context of binarization, the grayscale threshold T is chosen such that the total entropy $S = S_1 + S_2$ is maximized.

4.4.2 Connected Component Labeling

Binarization of the CT image by itself cannot represent distinctly the two fracture fragments, as is evident from Figs. 4.3(b) and 4.4(b). This is so because one still needs to filter out the undesired artifacts so that only the fractured mandibular fragments are used for the purpose of surface matching. A 2D Connected Component Labeling (CCL) procedure in conjunction with a component area filter was used to remove the undesired artifacts (which are typically small in size). The threshold value for the component area filter was chosen to be 1000 pixels. Connected components with area less than the threshold value were deleted. The result of these operations is illustrated in Figs. 4.3(c) and 4.4(c). The image processing tasks described thus far were performed on the individual 2D image slices comprising the CT image stack. The results of the 2D CCL were subsequently propagated across the CT image slices, resulting in a 3D CCL algorithm. A 3D component (a fractured mandibular bone fragment in this case) was identified by computing the area of overlap of the corresponding 2D components in successive CT image slices.

4.4.3 Contour Data Extraction

After performing the thresholding, CCL and size filtering operations on all the CT image slices, the task of interactive contour detection was performed on the resulting binary image slices. We used two approaches for this purpose. In one approach, the user is required to click on the end points of the fracture contours in each of the binary image slices. The intervening contour points are automatically generated using a contour tracing algorithm. In the other approach, the user can click on potentially interesting points on a fracture contour (typically points of high curvature).

In both approaches, the contour points obtained from the individual binary image slices were collated to generate the 3D surface point dataset. A 3D surface point dataset was generated for each fracture surface.

4.5 Surface Matching Using Type-0 Constraints

In this section, we describe two philosophically different algorithms, namely the ICP algorithm and the DARCES algorithm, for the purpose of registering the two broken bone fragments. We first employ the two algorithms individually and then in a synergistic manner. We denote the fracture surface (dataset) to be matched as the *sample* fracture surface (dataset) and the fracture surface (dataset) to which the sample fracture surface (dataset) is to be matched as the *model* fracture surface (dataset). The fragment containing the sample (model) fracture surface is denoted as the sample (model) fragment. The goal is to determine a (4×4) rigid body transformation from the matching of the sample and model fracture surfaces. This transformation is then applied to the entire sample fragment in order to register it with the entire model fragment. The term *type-0 constraints* implies the 3D coordinates of the points on the fracture surfaces. Thus, the fracture surfaces are matched based on the 3D coordinates (positions) of the constituent fracture surface points. Subsequently, we will show how *type-1 constraints* can be incorporated within the above registration procedure.

4.5.1 Surface Registration Using the ICP Algorithm

The ICP algorithm [47] is used to perform two tasks. The first task is to establish a correspondence between the two surface point sets to be matched. The second task is to compute the 3D transformation that brings the two sets into registration. In the context of our present problem, it is important to note that the cardinalities of the two datasets to be matched are different. The basic ICP algorithm consists of the following steps:

1. The matching points in the model dataset corresponding to points in the sample dataset are determined. This new set of matching points in the model dataset, which represents a subset of the original model dataset, is termed the *closest* set.
2. The 3D rigid body transformation (3D translation and 3D rotation) that brings the two surfaces into registration is computed. The transformation is obtained using the Theory of Quaternions [63].
3. The transformation thus computed is applied to the original sample dataset and the mean squared surface matching error (MSE) between the transformed sample data points and the corresponding closest points is calculated. The MSE (ϵ^2) is given by

$$\epsilon^2 = (1/n) \sum_{i=1}^{n} \left((c_i - (Rs_i + T))^2 \right), \tag{4.3}$$

where R denotes the rotation matrix, T denotes the translation vector, s_i denotes a point of the sample data set, c_i represents the corresponding point in the closest set, and n is the total number of sample points.

Steps 1–3 are repeated with an updated sample dataset (generated by applying R and T obtained in the current iteration to the current sample dataset) until the difference in MSE between two successive iterations drops below a prespecified threshold (0.01 mm^2 in our case).

We now discuss in detail the *closest set* computation, which is an important step in the ICP algorithm. Robust point matching remains a classical problem in the area of computer vision [64]. Graph-theoretic approaches have been used extensively in solving such problems [65]. In the computation of the closest set, which is the most crucial step in the ICP algorithm, the matching point pairs are determined using the Maximum Cardinality Minimum Weight (MCMW) bipartite graph matching algorithm based on the Hungarian method proposed by Kuhn [66]. We construct a bipartite graph $G(V_1 \cup V_2, E)$ where the 3D sample and model datasets correspond to the two disjoint vertex sets V_1 and V_2, respectively. The weight w_{ij} of an edge $e_{ij} \in E$ between two vertices v_i and v_j (where $v_i \in V_1$ and $v_j \in V_2$) is given by

$$w_{ij} = \left((x_i - x_j)^2 + (y_i - y_j)^2 + (z_i - z_j)^2\right)^{1/2}. \tag{4.4}$$

Invoking Theorem 2.2, we now state the following claim and provide an intuitive justification.

Claim 4.1 *Given that there is neither a reflection nor a very large* (*greater than* 90°) *rotation* (*two extremely unlikely cases for a typical craniofacial injury*), *the Maximum Cardinality Minimum Weight* (*MCMW*) *algorithm for a bipartite graph correctly establishes the correspondence between two fracture surfaces in each iteration of the Iterative Closest Point* (*ICP*) *algorithm in polynomial time.*

Justification Our justification is based on Theorem 2.2. Each fracture surface, consisting of several 3D data points, is modeled as a vertex set of a weighted bipartite graph $G = (V_1 \cup V_2, E)$. The bipartite graph is complete, i.e., there exists an edge $e_{ij} \in E$ between each vertex pair (v_i, v_j) where $v_i \in V_1$ and $v_j \in V_2$. The weight w_{ij} of edge e_{ij} is chosen to be the Euclidean distance between the corresponding vertices $v_i \in V_1$ and $v_j \in V_2$, where $i = 1, 2, \ldots, n_1 = |V_1|$, and $j = 1, 2, \ldots, n_2 = |V_2|$. The vertex set with lower cardinality is denoted as the *sample set*, and that with the higher cardinality is denoted as the *model set*. The goal is to compute the *closest set*, i.e., a maximal subset of the model set wherein each point corresponds to a unique point in the sample set such that all points in the sample set are exhausted (principle of maximum cardinality) and simultaneously the sum of the edge weights between all pairs of corresponding points (i.e., $\sum w_{ij}$) is minimized (principle of minimum weight). This procedure is carried out in each iteration of the ICP algorithm. In the absence of a reflection or a large (e.g., greater than 90°) rotation, this graph-theoretic optimization procedure, wherein the objective function is the *sum of the Euclidean distances between all pairs of matched points*, correctly matches a sample point with a model point without distorting the shape of the fracture surfaces. A greedy approach [35], based on the minimum Euclidean distance between individual pairs of points considered one at a time, on the other hand, could potentially map more than one sample point to a single model point and distort the fracture surface shape. Our problem formulation maps to the following well-known Maximum Cardinality Minimum Weight (MCMW) Bipartite Graph Matching Problem in graph theory, i.e., given a weighted complete bipartite graph $G = (V_1 \cup V_2, E)$ with edge-weights $w_{ij} \geq 0$, determine a pairing of the vertices from two vertex sets V_1 and V_2 such that the vertex set with smaller cardinality is completely exhausted and the total cost of the pairings is minimum. By virtue of its construction, the proposed bipartite graph is complete with $E = V_1 \times V_2$ where $|V_1| \leq |V_2|$ and such that there exists 1:1 mapping $f : V_1 \rightarrow V_2$. From Theorem 2.2, the MCMW algorithm runs in $O(n^3)$ time for a bipartite graph with two vertex sets of equal cardinality n. In our case, $n = \max(n_1, n_2)$. Thus, the proposed solution clearly runs in polynomial time. □

4.5.2 Registration Using the DARCES Algorithm

The DARCES algorithm [50] is used widely for solving 3D registration problems efficiently and reliably, especially in the presence of outliers. The DARCES algorithm does not require local feature detection or initial transformation estimation for the matching of two 3D data sets and thus differs from most feature-based approaches or iterative approaches to the 3D registration problem.

The main steps in the DARCES algorithm are as follows:

1. Reference points are selected from the sample data set. Note that the sample data set and the model data set have the same meaning as in the case of the ICP algorithm.
2. From the set of reference points three control points are chosen.
3. Based on certain predefined geometric constraints, the three corresponding matching points in the model data set are determined. Note that for the three control points, there are many such sets of three matching points in the model data set.
4. For each set of three pairs of corresponding points (i.e., the three control points and one set of three matched model points), a 3D rigid body transformation is obtained. Note that three pairs of corresponding points are sufficient to determine a 3D rigid body transformation.
5. Each transformation is then applied to all the reference points other than the three control points. If the distance between a transformed point and its nearest model point is below a certain threshold, then this reference point is considered to have been successfully aligned to the model surface. Thus, the number of successfully aligned sample data points is computed for each transformation.
6. The transformation which has successfully aligned the maximum number of sample data points is deemed to be the solution to the registration problem.

4.5.3 Registration Using the Hybrid DARCES–ICP Algorithm

We term the synergistic combination of the DARCES and ICP algorithm as the hybrid DARCES–ICP algorithm [53]. We begin with a claim and an intuitive justification that the hybrid DARCES–ICP algorithm would yield a lower mean squared surface matching error (MSE) when compared to the individual DARCES and ICP algorithms.

Claim 4.2 *The hybrid DARCES–ICP algorithm is expected to yield a lower MSE compared to that obtained by employing the DARCES and ICP algorithms individually.*

Justification The DARCES algorithm helps in outlier rejection, but the resulting transformation is only approximate. The ICP algorithm, on the other hand, yields a more accurate 3D rigid body transformation but is sensitive to outliers in the input data. Moreover, the pairs of matched points generated by the DARCES algorithm also helps in reducing the cardinalities of the two data sets to be matched (using MCMW Bipartite Graph Matching [33]) in the ICP algorithm. Thus, the relatively dense bipartite graph used to determine the closest set in the ICP algorithm can be reduced to a relatively sparse bipartite graph with fewer nodes and edges. The subsequent MCMW Bipartite Graph Matching Algorithm, (whose run time complexity is determined by the cardinalities of its vertex sets per Theorem 2.2) has a reduced computational complexity when run on a sparse bipartite graph. Simultaneously, a much lower MSE can be achieved for the matching of the two surfaces, since the DARCES algorithm provides a better starting point to the ICP algorithm by virtue of outlier removal. Thus, the synergistic combination of the DARCES and ICP algorithms, termed as hybrid DARCES–ICP algorithm (where the output of the DARCES algorithm is the input to the ICP algorithm), is expected to yield a higher reconstruction accuracy. □

We have exploited the synergism between the DARCES and ICP algorithms in the following three different ways [54]:

1. Using the DARCES transformed sample dataset and the model dataset as the two inputs to the ICP algorithm. Thus, the initial transformation estimate of the ICP algorithm is the one resulting from the DARCES algorithm. This is termed as *Synergism 1*.
2. Using a proper subset of the sample dataset (that has been aligned correctly by the DARCES algorithm) and the model dataset as the two inputs to the ICP algorithm. The initial transformation estimate used by the ICP algorithm is the default estimate, i.e., the initial rotation matrix is the identity matrix, and the initial translation vector is the null vector. This is termed as *Synergism 2*.
3. Using the DARCES transformed subset of the sample dataset and the model dataset as the two inputs to the ICP algorithm. Here, the proper subset of the sample dataset that has been aligned correctly by the DARCES algorithm is

used. Also, the initial transformation estimate of the ICP algorithm is the one resulting from the DARCES algorithm. This is tantamount to the combination of *Synergism 1* and *Synergism 2* and is termed as *Synergism 3*.

The composite transformation matrix $\theta_{\text{DARCES–ICP}}$ of the hybrid DARCES–ICP algorithm (consisting of a rotation matrix and a translation vector), to be applied to the sample dataset in order to register it with the model dataset is given by

$$[\theta_{\text{DARCES–ICP}}] = [\theta_{\text{DARCES}}][\theta_{\text{ICP}}], \tag{4.5}$$

where θ_{DARCES} and θ_{ICP} respectively denote the composite transformations obtained from the individual DARCES and ICP algorithms.

4.6 Improved Surface Matching with Surface Irregularity Modeling

We have, thus far, treated all points on a fracture surface on an equal footing. Our next goal is to classify and label the individual discrete sampled points on the two opposable fracture surfaces and incorporate the classification and labeling information in our reconstruction paradigm to further improve the reconstruction accuracy [55]. We employ two different approaches for this purpose. The first approach categorizes the fracture surface points into various primitive surface categories based on the signs of the local mean (H) and Gaussian (K) surface curvature values. The second approach uses the theory of fuzzy sets to model the surface irregularities. The classification and labeling information is exploited during the determination of correspondence between the points on the two fracture surfaces using various reward–penalty schemes.

4.6.1 Curvature-Based Surface Irregularity Estimation

There exist techniques in the literature for feature classification based on surface labeling of voxels or pixels in volumetric images [67]. Typically, the digital surface, within a local window, is approximated by an analytic surface using a least-squares surface fitting technique [68–70]. In our case, discrete biorthogonal Chebyshev polynomials [68, 71] are used as the basis functions in a local $N \times N$ window (where $N = 5$ in our case) around each surface point to compute the local H and K values. We follow the notation of [68] for the remainder of this section. The elements of the First Fundamental Form matrix $\mathbf{G}$ of the surface can be expressed in terms of the estimates of the first-order partial derivatives f_u and f_v of the surface function $f(u, v)$ as follows:

$$\begin{aligned} g_{11} &= 1 + f_u^2, \\ g_{22} &= 1 + f_v^2, \\ g_{12} &= g_{21} = f_u f_v. \end{aligned} \tag{4.6}$$

Similarly, the elements of the Second Fundamental Form matrix **B** of the surface can be expressed in terms of the estimates of the aforementioned first-order partial derivatives and the second-order partial derivatives f_{uu}, f_{vv}, and f_{uv} of the surface function $f(u, v)$ as follows:

$$\begin{aligned} b_{11} &= f_{uu}/\sqrt{1+f_u^2+f_v^2}, \\ b_{22} &= f_{vv}/\sqrt{1+f_u^2+f_v^2}, \\ b_{12} = b_{21} &= f_{uv}/\sqrt{1+f_u^2+f_v^2}. \end{aligned} \tag{4.7}$$

The digital surface is approximated using discrete biorthogonal Chebyshev polynomials [69]. As mentioned before, discrete biorthogonal Chebyshev polynomials are used as basis functions in a local $N \times N$ window (where N is odd) centered about the point of interest (u, v). Thus, each data point in a given $N \times N$ window is associated with a position (u, v) from the set $U \times U$, where

$$U = \left\{ \frac{-(N-1)}{2}, \ldots, -1, 0, 1, \ldots, \frac{(N-1)}{2} \right\}. \tag{4.8}$$

A surface function estimate $\hat{f}(u, v)$ is obtained of the form

$$\hat{f}(u, v) = \sum_{i=0}^{2} \sum_{j=0}^{2} a_{ij} \phi_i(u) \phi_j(v) \tag{4.9}$$

that minimizes the total squared error term

$$\varepsilon^2 = \sum_{(u,v) \in U \times U} \left(f(u, v) - \hat{f}(u, v) \right)^2. \tag{4.10}$$

The solution for the unknown coefficients a_{ij} is given by

$$a_{ij} = \sum_{(u,v) \in U \times U} f(u, v) \psi_i(u) \psi_j(v). \tag{4.11}$$

Here the $\psi_i' s$ are the normalized versions of the orthogonal Chebyshev polynomials ϕ_i and are given by

$$\begin{aligned} \psi_0(u) &= \frac{1}{N}, \\ \psi_1(u) &= \left(\frac{3}{M(M+1)(2M+1)} \right) u, \\ \psi_2(u) &= \frac{1}{P(M)} \left(u^2 - \frac{M(M+1)}{3} \right), \end{aligned} \tag{4.12}$$

where $M = \frac{(N-1)}{2}$, and $P(M)$ is the fifth-order polynomial in M given by

$$P(M) = \frac{8}{45} M^5 + \frac{4}{9} M^4 + \frac{2}{9} M^3 - \frac{1}{9} M^2 - \frac{1}{15} M. \tag{4.13}$$

Table 4.1 Classification of surface pixels based on the signs of the H and K values [71]

H, K	$H < 0$	$H = 0$	$H > 0$
$K < 0$	Saddle Ridge	Minimal Surface	Saddle Valley
$K = 0$	Ridge Surface	Flat Surface	Valley Surface
$K > 0$	Peak Surface	None	Pit Surface

The coefficients a_{ij} of the functional approximation are computed using equations (4.11)–(4.13). The first- and second-order partial derivatives of the fitted surface are given in terms of the $a'_{ij}s$ as follows:

$$\begin{aligned} f_u &= a_{10}, \\ f_v &= a_{01}, \\ f_{uv} &= a_{11}, \\ f_{uu} &= 2a_{20}, \\ f_{vv} &= 2a_{02}. \end{aligned} \tag{4.14}$$

The elements of **G** and **B** are estimated next using (4.6) and (4.7). The principal curvatures (κ_1, κ_2) are found to be the roots of the following quadratic equation [70]:

$$|\mathbf{G}|\kappa_n^2 - (g_{11}b_{22} + b_{11}g_{22} - 2g_{12}b_{12})\kappa_n + |\mathbf{B}| = 0, \quad n = 1, 2, \tag{4.15}$$

where $|\mathbf{G}|$ and $|\mathbf{B}|$ denote the magnitudes of the determinants of matrices **G** and **B**, respectively.

The mean and Gaussian curvatures can be respectively expressed in terms of the principal curvatures (κ_1, κ_2) as follows:

$$\begin{aligned} H &= (\kappa_1 + \kappa_2)/2 = (g_{11}b_{22} + g_{22}b_{11} - 2g_{12}b_{12})/2\left(g_{11}g_{22} - g_{12}^2\right), \\ K &= \kappa_1\kappa_2 = \left(b_{11}b_{22} - b_{12}^2\right)/\left(g_{11}g_{22} - g_{12}^2\right). \end{aligned} \tag{4.16}$$

The signs of H and K are used to classify the surface point into one of eight qualitative surface types (see Table 4.1). The above procedure is repeated for each point on each of the fracture surfaces for which a valid local window exists.

4.6.2 Fuzzy Set Theory-Based Surface Irregularity Extraction

We have also investigated an alternative approach based on fuzzy set theory to categorize the sampled points on the fracture surfaces. Two fuzzy sets termed as *droop* and *bulge* are formulated to classify these points [72]. Fuzzy set theory not only permits us to classify a contour point as a droop or a bulge, but also enables us to specify the extent of this droop or bulge. The average variation of the fracture surface in a direction perpendicular to the plane of fracture is estimated and is denoted by $\bar{x}$. Note that a fracture surface consists of several fracture contours. For each point on each such contour, the deviation from the average, i.e., $(p_x - \bar{x})$ is determined, where p_x is the x coordinate of a point p. If $p_x > \bar{x}$, then the point p is deemed to belong to the *bulge* fuzzy set, else it is deemed to belong to the *droop* fuzzy set. The goal here is to highlight the surface irregularity and subsequently be able to discriminate between the surface points on the basis of their fuzzy membership values. The fuzzy membership function used for surface labeling is given by

$$\mu_{\text{droop/bulge}} = 1 - \exp\bigl(-k|p_x - \bar{x}|\bigr), \tag{4.17}$$

where $\mu_{\text{droop/bulge}}$ is the membership value of a point p (with x coordinate value p_x) in the fuzzy set *droop* or *bulge*, as the case may be. The constant k for a particular contour is determined by setting $\mu_{\text{droop/bulge}}$ to be very close to 1 (e.g., 0.99) and using the maximum value of $(|p_x - \bar{x}|)$ for all the points on that contour. This approach for determining the value of k takes into consideration, very precisely, the local variations of the surface coordinate values, with respect to the global average of the surface coordinate values over the entire fracture surface. The above fuzzy classification procedure is performed for all points on each of the fracture surfaces.

4.6.3 Reward/Penalty Schemes

Two reward/penalty schemes are introduced to emphasize the effect of the extracted surface irregularities on the process of establishing faithful correspondence between the opposing fracture surfaces. Note that each pair of corresponding points on the opposing fracture surfaces is represented by the corresponding elements of the two vertex sets of a bipartite graph. With the incorporation of reward/penalty schemes, the original edge weights w_{ij} between the two corresponding points i and j are modified by the introduction of a reward–penalty term RP_{ij}. The new edge weights w'_{ij} are given by

$$w'_{ij} = w_{ij} + \lambda RP_{ij}, \tag{4.18}$$

where λ is termed as the reward–penalty coefficient. The use of two distinct methods to determine the term RP_{ij} is consistent with the two different methods employed for surface feature extraction. A *binary reward/penalty* scheme is adopted in the case of curvature-based surface classification, and a *fuzzy reward/penalty* scheme is chosen in the case of fuzzy set theory-based surface classification.

In the case of the *binary reward/penalty* approach, the signs of the mean and Gaussian curvature values H and K for a pair of corresponding points from the two opposing fracture surfaces are examined. Accordingly, a value is assigned to the reward/penalty term RP_{ij} for this pair based on Table 4.2. The value of RP_{ij} is 1 in case of a reward and -1 in case of a penalty. If there exists no proper local window surrounding a point, then it is not classified into a primitive surface category based on the signs of H and K, i.e., the point is deemed as unclassified. A pair of points in which at least one of the points is unclassified is not assigned a reward or penalty value.

Table 4.2 Assignment of reward–penalty value based on the signs of the H, K values for any two surface points

Two points i, j	RP_{ij}
Saddle Ridge, Saddle Valley	−1.0
Ridge Surface, Valley Surface	−1.0
Flat Surface, Flat Surface	−1.0
Peak Surface, Pit Surface	−1.0
At least one unclassified point	0.0
All other cases	1.0

In the case of the *fuzzy reward/penalty* approach, two separate fuzzy functions, $\mu_R(\mu_i, \mu_j)$ and $\mu_P(\mu_i, \mu_j)$, are designed to quantify the reward and the penalty, respectively. If the two points within a pair of corresponding points belong to the same fuzzy set, then they receive a penalty, else they receive a reward. The need for two distinct functions stems from the fact that the reward is *inversely* proportional to the difference in membership values, whereas the penalty is *directly* proportional to the difference in membership values. The fuzzy reward function μ_R for two points i and j is a function of the individual membership values μ_i and μ_j of these two points in the fuzzy sets *droop* and *bulge*, respectively, and is given by the following equation:

$$\mu_R(\mu_i, \mu_j) = 2/\big(1 + \exp\big(r_c|\mu_i - \mu_j|\big)\big), \tag{4.19}$$

where r_c is the reward constant. The value of r_c is chosen such that μ_R is close to 0 when $|\mu_i - \mu_j|$ is maximum (i.e., $= 1$). We used the following equation to estimate r_c:

$$0.01 = 2/\big(1 + \exp(r_c)\big). \tag{4.20}$$

The fuzzy penalty function μ_P for two points i and j is also a function of the individual membership values μ_i and μ_j of these two points in the fuzzy sets *droop* and *bulge*, respectively, and is given by the following equation:

$$\mu_P(\mu_i, \mu_j) = 1 - \exp\big(-p_c|\mu_i - \mu_j|\big), \tag{4.21}$$

where p_c is the penalty constant. The value of p_c is chosen such that μ_P is close to 1 when $|\mu_i - \mu_j|$ is maximum (i.e., $= 1$). We used the following equation to estimate p_c:

$$0.99 = 1 - \exp(-p_c). \tag{4.22}$$

4.7 Improved Surface Matching with Type-1 Constraints

The primary motivation behind the hybrid DARCES–ICP algorithm is to improve the performance of the ICP algorithm. The DARCES algorithm helps in the rejection of outliers and serves to initialize the ICP algorithm with a sparser and more accurate set of corresponding points from the opposing fracture surfaces. However, it is important to note that in the 3D surface registration procedure we have thus far limited ourselves to *type-0* constraints, i.e., the matching of corresponding points on the opposing fracture surfaces is based solely on the Euclidean distance between their 3D coordinate values and their individual local surface characteristics. It is quite logical to exploit, within the registration paradigm, additional geometric information or constraints of a relational nature, which we term as *type-1* constraints. First, we generate multiple initial solutions for the ICP algorithm based on certain relational geometric constraints. Next, we identify the best initial candidate solution for the surface registration problem. Finally, we propose another hybrid surface registration algorithm and term it the Geometric-ICP algorithm [56, 57].

4.7.1 Cycle Graph Automorphs as Initial ICP States

Besl and McKay [47] have suggested multiple initializations as a means to attain a global minimum in their version of the ICP algorithm. They have suggested comparing shape-based principal moments and sampling the quaternion states based on rotation groups of regular polyhedra to produce multiple initial starting states for the ICP algorithm. We have chosen to generate multiple solutions, one of which is to be eventually used as the starting point for the ICP algorithm, based on the automorphism group of the bounding box of a fracture surface which is modeled as a cycle graph. The bounding box for a single fracture surface is constructed simply by using two pairs of extreme points of a fracture contour that appear in the first and last image slice of the CT image sequence. The bounding box is modeled as a cycle graph of order 4. Note that the bounding box of a fracture surface can be replaced by its convex hull to yield a more general model of the fracture surface. The weights assigned to the edges of the cycle graph are the Euclidean distances between the corresponding points. The main idea is that if the two fracture surfaces are well matched, then their corresponding bounding boxes are also well matched. From Theorem 2.4, a cycle graph of order 4 has 8 automorphs. Thus, we have a total of 8 initial states, where each initial state is an automorph of the bounding box of one of the fracture surfaces.

4.7.2 Selection of the Best Initial State

Note that the MCMW bipartite graph matching algorithm essentially establishes the correspondence between the points on the two opposable fracture surfaces. We show how *type-1* constraints and knowledge of global shape can be used to improve the results of the surface registration procedure. Kim and Kak [65] have shown how local *type-0* and *type-1* geometric constraints can be exploited to improve the correspondence between two feature sets in the context of object recognition. We introduce a dissimilarity function based on *type-1* constraints that are invariant to rigid body transformation. Let us denote the cycle graph of the fracture surface of one broken mandibular fragment *frg*$_1$ by B_1, and that of the other broken mandibular fragment *frg*$_2$ by B_2. Let AB_2 denote the set of automorphs of B_2 and $AB_{2,l}$ the lth automorph of B_2. In order for B_1 and $AB_{2,l}$ to be well matched:

1. The lengths of corresponding pairs of sides of B_1 and $AB_{2,l}$ should be well matched. Let us denote the lengths of the ith sides of B_1 and $AB_{2,l}$ by d_i^1 and $d_i^{2,l}$, respectively.
2. The angles between the corresponding pairs of sides of B_1 and $AB_{2,l}$ should also be well matched. Let us denote the angle bounded by sides i and j of B_1 and $AB_{2,l}$ by $\theta_{i,j}^1$ and $\theta_{i,j}^{2,l}$, respectively.

Let the four vertices of B_1 and $AB_{2,l}$ be denoted by $(v_1^1, \ldots, v_4^1)$ and $(v_1^{2,l}, \ldots, v_4^{2,l})$. Each vertex can be considered a point in 3D space, e.g., v_1^1 has coordinates xv_1^1, yv_1^1, zv_1^1, and so on. Then d_i^k (where $k = 1, (2, l)$ and $i = 1, \ldots, 4$) is given by

$$d_i^k = \Big[\big(xv_i^k - xv_{((i \bmod 4)+1)}^k\big)^2 + \big(yv_i^k - yv_{((i \bmod 4)+1)}^k\big)^2 + \big(zv_i^k - zv_{((i \bmod 4)+1)}^k\big)^2\Big]^{1/2}. \tag{4.23}$$

Likewise, $\theta_{i,j}^k$ (where $k = 1, (2, l)$, $i = 1, \ldots, 4$ and $j = 1, \ldots, 4$) can be written as

$$\theta_{i,j}^k = \arccos\big((\mathbf{d}_\mathbf{i}^\mathbf{k} \cdot \mathbf{d}_\mathbf{j}^\mathbf{k})/(|\mathbf{d}_\mathbf{i}^\mathbf{k}||\mathbf{d}_\mathbf{j}^\mathbf{k}|)\big). \tag{4.24}$$

The dissimilarity function $\Gamma(B_1, AB_{2,l})$ between B_1 and the lth member of AB_2 can now be defined as a linear combination of the above factors:

$$\begin{aligned} \Gamma(B_1, AB_{2,l}) &= \lambda_1 \Gamma_1(B_1, AB_{2,l}) + \lambda_2 \Gamma_2(B_1, AB_{2,l}), \quad \text{where} \\ \Gamma_1(B_1, AB_{2,l}) &= \sum_{i=1}^{4} \big(|d_i^1 - d_i^{2,l}|\big), \text{ and} \\ \Gamma_2(B_1, AB_{2,l}) &= \sum_{i=1}^{4} \big(|\theta_{i,((i \bmod 4)+1)}^1 - \theta_{i,((i \bmod 4)+1)}^{2,l}|\big). \end{aligned} \tag{4.25}$$

The values of λ_1 and λ_2 are determined from the variations of the terms $\Gamma_1(B_1, AB_{2,l})$ and $\Gamma_2(B_1, AB_{2,l})$ for the 8 possible values of l and from the normalization constraint $\lambda_1 + \lambda_2 = 1$. The dissimilarity function $\Gamma(B_1, AB_{2,l})$ is computed between B_1 and each of the automorphs in AB_2. The lower the value of the dissimilarity function $\Gamma(B_1, AB_{2,l})$, the better the match between B_1 and $AB_{2,l}$. The 8 automorphs are ranked in ascending order of their $\Gamma(B_1, AB_{2,l})$ values and the first 4 automorphs are chosen as the most suitable candidates for being opposable to B_1.

Next, we exploit global shape knowledge for the extraction of the best initial solution from the 4 highest ranking automorphs. After the four members of AB_2 that yield the lowest $\Gamma(B_1, AB_{2,l})$ values have been determined, the corresponding four transformations $(\phi_1, \ldots, \phi_4)$ between B_1 and the eligible automorphs are estimated. Each of these four transformations is then applied to *frg*$_1$ to register it to *frg*$_2$. Wang et al. [58] have used geodesics and local geometry to improve the surface correspondence. In our case, we apply knowledge of the global shape of the human mandible to disambiguate between the four reconstructed mandibles by comparing them with an intact reference mandible using a suitable shape similarity measure. The contours $Co_1, \ldots, Co_4$ of each of the reconstructed mandibles and contour Co_{ref} of the intact reference mandible are extracted using simple edge detection. Contour-based shape similarity measures have been well explored in the computer vision literature (e.g., see [73]). We have chosen the Hausdorff distance for the present problem because of its relatively low $O(n^2)$ computational complexity and because it circumvents the need to establish prior correspondence between the pixels of the two contours under consideration. The bounding box for each of the five contours is determined. Each contour is scaled to ensure that its bounding box fits the input image exactly. The Contour Hausdorff Distance (CHD) between two scaled contour data sets Co_i (where $i = 1, \ldots, 4$) and Co_{ref} is given by [74]:

$$H(Co_i, Co_{\text{ref}}) = \max\big(h(Co_i, Co_{\text{ref}}), h(Co_{\text{ref}}, Co_i)\big), \tag{4.26}$$

where $h(Co_i, Co_{\text{ref}})$ is the directed Hausdorff distance between the two data sets Co_i and Co_{ref} and is defined as

$$h(Co_i, Co_{\text{ref}}) = \max_{a \in Co_i} \min_{b \in Co_{\text{ref}}} \|a - b\|. \tag{4.27}$$

Here $\|a - b\|$ represents the Euclidean distance between the points a and b. The contour Co^* that yields the minimum value of CHD is deemed to be the best matching contour, and the corresponding transformation ϕ^* is treated as the best initial state for the ICP algorithm. We term the above coarse registration approach as the *Geometric* algorithm.

4.7.3 Registration Using the Hybrid Geometric–ICP Algorithm

The transformation ϕ^* generated by the Geometric algorithm is used as the initial transformation for the ICP algorithm. The ICP algorithm initialized with ϕ^* is termed the *Geometric–ICP* algorithm. It is expected that the Geometric–ICP (GICP) algorithm, on account of better initialization, should result in lower surface registration error. The transformation ϕ_{GICP} of the Geometric–ICP algorithm can be also interpreted as the following composite transformation:

$$[\phi_{\text{GICP}}] = [\phi^*][\phi_{\text{ICP}}], \tag{4.28}$$

where ϕ_{ICP} denotes the transformation obtained using the conventional ICP algorithm. We also measure the MSE resulting from the best possible coarse registration transformation ϕ^* computed using the Geometric algorithm. It is important to realize that although the Geometric algorithm exploits geometric constraints and knowledge of global shape, it uses only four pairs of corresponding points and lacks the iterative refinement capability of the ICP algorithm. Note that (4.28) is similar to (4.5) where the input to the ICP algorithm comes from the Geometric algorithm in one case and from the DARCES algorithm in the other.

4.8 Bilateral Symmetry of the Human Mandible

The surface matching algorithms discussed thus far are mostly surface data-driven and, to a large extent, local in their scope. The surface matching algorithms described in Sect. 4.5 satisfied only the *type-0* constraints by matching the corresponding points on the two fracture surfaces. The use of *type-1* constraints and global shape knowledge was explored in Sect. 4.7. To ensure a more accurate preservation of the global shape of the reconstructed mandible, symmetry issues are considered next. There exists extensive research literature [75–77] in the areas of mathematics, computer vision, and image processing, dealing with different types of symmetry such as reflection symmetry, rotation symmetry, and skew symmetry. Anatomical knowledge of the human mandible clearly demonstrates the presence of bilateral or reflection symmetry. The mathematical notion of reflection symmetry is introduced next following the mathematical notation in [78].

Let $\mathbf{m}$ be a unit vector in 3D space $\mathbf{R}^3$, S^2 the unit sphere of all possible directions in $\mathbf{R}^3$, and $\mathbf{\Pi}_{\mathbf{m},n}$ a plane in $\mathbf{R}^3$ orthogonal to the vector $\mathbf{m}$ and passing at distance n from the origin. Let $\mathbf{g}$ be any image with its elements denoted as $\mathbf{g}(x,y,z)$, and $\mathbf{h} = e_{\mathbf{m},n}(g)$ be the reflected image with respect to the plane $\mathbf{\Pi}_{\mathbf{m},n}$, with elements given by $\mathbf{h}(x,y,z)$. Then, we can state

$$e_{\mathbf{m},n}\big(\mathbf{g}(x,y,z)\big) = \mathbf{g}\big(e_{\mathbf{m},n}(x,y,z)\big).$$

The image $\mathbf{g}$ is called *reflection symmetrical* if there exists a reflection plane $\mathbf{\Pi}_{\mathbf{m},n}$ such that $\mathbf{h} = \mathbf{g}$. In such a case, $\mathbf{\Pi}_{\mathbf{m},n}$ will be a plane of reflection symmetry for $\mathbf{g}$. Our goal is to find the plane of maximal bilateral symmetry with respect to some appropriate symmetry measure $\psi(\mathbf{g},\mathbf{h})$. It is well known that the planes of reflection symmetry of any rigid body pass through its center of mass and are orthogonal to the axes of the ellipsoid of inertia [79]. The moment of inertia matrix M of a rigid body is given by

$$\begin{pmatrix} \mu_{200} & \mu_{110} & \mu_{101} \\ \mu_{110} & \mu_{020} & \mu_{011} \\ \mu_{101} & \mu_{011} & \mu_{002} \end{pmatrix}.$$

The elements of the 3×3 moment of inertia matrix M are the second-order centralized moments for the rigid body under consideration. Thus, each matrix element μ_{pqr} can be written as

$$\mu_{pqr} = \iiint f(x,y,z)(x-x_c)^p(y-y_c)^q(z-z_c)^r\,dx\,dy\,dz. \tag{4.29}$$

In (4.29), (x_c, y_c, z_c) denotes the coordinates of the centroid of the mandible, each of the powers p, q, and r can assume any value between 0 and 2, and $f(x,y,z)$ is the mass distribution function. For the segmented mandible, $f(x,y,z)$ is binary, i.e., we can write

$$f(x,y,z) = \begin{cases} 1 & \text{if } (x,y,z) \in \text{mandible}, \\ 0 & \text{otherwise.} \end{cases} \tag{4.30}$$

In this case, we can drop the $f(x,y,z)$ term from the integrand in (4.29). The eigenvalues of M are obtained from the roots of the secular equation [80]. Since the secular equation is cubic, there are three possible eigenvalues and three corresponding eigenvectors. Thus, the number of potential candidates for the plane of reflection symmetry is restricted to three. This obviates the need for an exhaustive search for determining the plane of symmetry. We express the plane of reflection symmetry $\boldsymbol{\Pi}_{\mathbf{m},n}$ using the general equation of a three-dimensional plane as in [81, 82]:

$$F(x, y, z) = ax + by + cz - d = 0. \tag{4.31}$$

In (4.31), (a, b, c) is a vector describing the normal to the plane. The perpendicular distance of the plane from the origin is given by $d/\sqrt{a^2 + b^2 + c^2}$. Once the coefficients of the three planes of symmetry are determined, the entire mandible is reflected about each of the three planes. To obtain the desired plane of bilateral symmetry, we compute the following:

$$\max\big(\psi(\mathbf{g}, \mathbf{h}_1), \psi(\mathbf{g}, \mathbf{h}_2), \psi(\mathbf{g}, \mathbf{h}_3)\big),$$

where $\mathbf{h}_1, \mathbf{h}_2, \mathbf{h}_3$ represent the three reflected mandibles, and $\mathbf{g}$ the reconstructed mandible. For each voxel $\mathbf{g}(x, y, z)$ in the reconstructed mandible $\mathbf{g}$, there exists a corresponding $\mathbf{h}(x, y, z)$ in each of the reflected mandibles $\mathbf{h}$ (where $\mathbf{h} \in \{\mathbf{h}_1, \mathbf{h}_2, \mathbf{h}_3\}$) which can be estimated using the following equation [82]:

$$\mathbf{h}(x, y, z) = \begin{cases} \mathbf{g}(x, y, z) - \frac{F(\mathbf{g})}{\|\nabla F\|} \frac{\nabla F}{\|\nabla F\|} & \text{if } F(x, y, z) > 0, \\ \mathbf{g}(x, y, z) + \frac{F(\mathbf{g})}{\|\nabla F\|} \frac{\nabla F}{\|\nabla F\|} & \text{otherwise,} \end{cases} \tag{4.32}$$

where $F(x, y, z)$ is computed using (4.31). There are various measures of symmetry described in the research literature [78, 83, 84] such as the sum of absolute distance, sum of squared distance, and normalized cross-correlation. Of these various measures, we have chosen the normalized cross-correlation to quantify the extent of symmetry $\psi(\mathbf{g}, \mathbf{h})$. The normalized cross-correlation between the reconstructed mandible $\mathbf{g}$ and the reflected mandible $\mathbf{h}$, where $\mathbf{g}$ and $\mathbf{h}$ are each represented by a K-dimensional vector, is given by [82]

$$\psi(\mathbf{g}, \mathbf{h}) = \frac{(\mathbf{g} - \overline{g}\mathbf{u})(\mathbf{h} - \overline{h}\mathbf{u})}{\|(\mathbf{g} - \overline{g}\mathbf{u})\| \, \|\mathbf{h} - \overline{h}\mathbf{u})\|}, \tag{4.33}$$

where $\overline{g}$ and $\overline{h}$ are the means of the elements of $\mathbf{g}$ and $\mathbf{h}$, respectively, and $\mathbf{u}$ is a K-dimensional unit vector. Of the three candidate planes of symmetry, the one about which the corresponding reflected mandible yields the maximum value of the symmetry measure, is deemed as the plane of bilateral or reflection symmetry. The corresponding symmetry measure is deemed as the coefficient of symmetry. It should be noted that our principal aim is the computation of the coefficient of symmetry rather than very accurate determination of the plane of symmetry. Thus, we have not employed a sophisticated optimization technique such as the Downhill Simplex method [80] to further refine the coefficients of the plane of bilateral symmetry.

4.9 Biomechanical Stability of the Human Mandible

Since the human mandible is a solid body with known biomechanical properties, we next evaluate the biomechanical stability of the reconstructed mandible. It is critical for the reconstructed mandible to be biomechanically stable so that it can withstand the stresses resulting from the normal masticatory function of the human jaw. We first present a validation of our claim that maximizing the biomechanical stability of a 3D rigid object, under certain conditions, is tantamount to minimizing its surface area. Next, we present techniques from 3D differential geometry to actually compute the surface area. Once again, the goal is to improve the overall reconstruction process by inclusion of a biomechanical stability criterion. We now state and justify the following claim:

Claim 4.3 *Maximum biomechanical stability of a rigid linear body under conditions of near zero volumetric response and constant surface force is ensured by a state with minimum surface area.*

Justification A biomechanically stable state for a rigid 3D body with linear material (stress–strain) properties can be conceived as a state with minimum potential energy U. The general form of U is given by [85]

$$U = \iiint f(\varphi, \chi, Y, \sigma)\, dv,$$

where φ, χ, Y, and σ denote the normal strain, shear strain, Young's Modulus, and Poisson ratio, respectively. Let us consider a deformed body with volume V, surface area S, a volume load (basically body force) B, and surface load (basically shear force)!T. Then U can be mathematically expressed in a way similar to that in [86]:

$$U = \iiint L_b(u)\, dv + \iint L_s(u)\, ds, \tag{4.34}$$

where $L_b(u)$ and $L_s(u)$ respectively denote the volume load potential and surface load potential, and u is the displacement field. The potential functions $L_b(u)$ and $L_s(u)$ are related to the body force B and shear force T as follows:

$$\begin{aligned} B &= -\frac{\delta L_b(u)}{\delta u}, \\ T &= -\frac{\delta L_s(u)}{\delta u}. \end{aligned} \tag{4.35}$$

Applying the calculus of variations to (4.34) and using (4.35), we obtain

$$\delta U = \iiint [-B \cdot \delta u]\, dV + \iint [-T \cdot \delta u]\, dS. \tag{4.36}$$

The normal and shear strains occurring in response to a force field are represented by the displacement field u and resisted by forces arising from the Young's and shear moduli. The body force B and the surface shear forces T will result in a deformation pattern that minimizes U. From (4.36) we can state that the following criterion must be satisfied under equilibrium conditions:

$$\iint [-T \cdot \delta u]\, dS + \iiint [-B \cdot \delta u]\, dV - \delta U = 0. \tag{4.37}$$

For the purpose of this discussion, we may assume near zero resistance to movement resulting from a force of unity. Thus, the energy related to the volumetric response, i.e., the second term in (4.37), is near zero. Hence, it can be concluded that a minimum potential energy state results in minimum surface energy. Further, minimum surface energy in the context of moving fragments with constant surface force T (which makes the quantity within the square bracket in the first term in (4.37) a constant) is consistent with minimum surface area (leaving $\|\delta U\| \propto \iint dS$). Thus, a biomechanically stable state (i.e., a state with minimum potential energy) is guaranteed by a state with minimum surface area. □

Since, the human mandible possesses curved surfaces, we employ techniques from differential geometry to compute the surface area. A digital surface S can be parameterized as $\mathbf{S}(u, v) = (u, v, f(u, v))$. The area A of surface S can be written as [68]

$$A = \iint \sqrt{g}\, du\, dv, \tag{4.38}$$

where g is the *metric determinant* defined as the determinant of the *First Fundamental Form* matrix $\mathbf{G}$) of the surface S, i.e., $g = |\mathbf{G}|$ [70]. We divide the surface S into an appropriate number (say n) of disjoint surface patches where SP_i denotes the ith surface patch with an associated *metric determinant* g_i. Thus, we obtain:

$$\begin{aligned} S &= \bigcup_{i=1}^{n} SP_i, \\ SP_i \cap SP_j &= \Phi \quad \text{if } i \neq j, \end{aligned} \tag{4.39}$$

where Φ is a null set. Based on the above, we can modify (4.38) as

$$\begin{aligned} A &= \sum_{i=1}^{n} A_i, \\ \text{where } A_i &= \iint \sqrt{g_i}\, du\, dv. \end{aligned} \tag{4.40}$$

4.10 Composite Reconstruction Using MSE, Symmetry, and Stability

The various reconstruction algorithms, described earlier in the chapter, dealt exclusively with the accuracy of registration of the two fracture surfaces under consideration. Thus, the symmetry and the biomechanical stability constraints cannot be explicitly enforced in the first phase of the reconstruction. In this section, we first introduce a composite reconstruction metric containing all the three factors, i.e., registration accuracy, shape symmetry, and biomechanical stability. We propose a simple, yet effective, scheme to minimize this metric.

The principal rationale behind the second phase of reconstruction, which consists of an angular perturbation scheme, is to arrive at a configuration that not only minimizes the MSE between the matched fracture surfaces but also results in the best possible shape symmetry and biomechanical stability of the reconstructed mandible. A composite reconstruction metric (*CRM*), expressed as a linear combination of three terms, i.e., the MSE, global shape symmetry, and biomechanical stability, is proposed as the overall performance measure of the two-phase virtual reconstruction paradigm. The *CRM* is treated as the objective function of a convex optimization problem. The *inverse* of the symmetry measure $\psi(\mathbf{g}, \mathbf{h})$ (4.33) is included as one of the terms in the *CRM* since the *CRM* optimization problem is cast as one of minimization. Thus, the goal is to obtain a reconstruction of the fractured mandible which results in minimum MSE, minimum value of the inverse of the symmetry measure, and minimum surface area (shown to be a measure of biomechanical stability per Claim 4.3). Mathematically, the *CRM* is given by [60]

$$\Omega = \lambda_1 \epsilon^2 + \lambda_2 \psi^{-1} + \lambda_3 \bar{A}, \tag{4.41}$$

where the MSE (ϵ^2) is computed using (4.3), the inverse of the shape symmetry ψ^{-1} is estimated using (4.33), and the average surface area $\bar{A}$ is determined using (4.40).

There exist several standard algorithms for convex optimization problems [80]. However, we have chosen to use a small-scale angular perturbation scheme to optimize the proposed *CRM*. Our strategy is to recompute each of the three terms in (4.41) for all possible reconstruction states generated for a range of suitably quantized angular perturbations about each of the three principal X, Y, and Z axes. A similar optimization strategy can be found in [16]. Essentially, we need a fine refinement ϕ_{AP} of the basic transformation obtained from any of the ICP, DARCES, hybrid DARCES–ICP, and hybrid Geometric–ICP algorithms. In our case, we have applied the angular perturbation scheme to the result of the hybrid DARCES–ICP algorithm. It is assumed that ϕ_{AP} consists of a small angular rotation and no translation. The composite transformation (ϕ_{Comp}) of the two-phase reconstruction procedure can be expressed in terms of the transformation $\phi_{\mathrm{DARCES–ICP}}$ obtained from the hybrid DARCES–ICP algorithm and the transformation ϕ_{AP} obtained from the angular perturbation scheme as follows:

$$[\phi_{\mathrm{Comp}}] = [\phi_{\mathrm{AP}}][\phi_{\mathrm{DARCES–ICP}}]. \tag{4.42}$$

Typically, ϕ_{AP} is a combination of clockwise or counterclockwise rotations about the three principal X, Y, and Z axes. The range and quantization of angular perturbation are based on heuristics and a trade-off between accuracy and computational complexity. Since we have already achieved a locally good solution (i.e., one that represents a local minimum of the MSE) in the first phase of the reconstruction, we can make a heuristic argument that this locally good solution is not very far off from the best overall solution (i.e., one resulting in the minimum Ω value). This heuristic provides a rationale for why we do not need a sophisticated optimization technique and subsequently allows us to limit the range of angular perturbations. The choice of the angular quantization represents a judicious trade-off between the execution time and the desired accuracy of the final reconstruction. The smaller the angular quantization, the higher the computational complexity (and execution time) of the reconstruction algorithm. On the other hand, a too large angular quantization may prevent the reconstruction algorithm from arriving at the best possible solution and thereby compromise the accuracy of the final reconstruction. Additionally, we are also interested in determining whether the MSE by itself could be reduced any further. The aforementioned angular perturbation approach, in its search for the lowest *CRM* value via exploration of the reconstruction states that are rotationally close to the one obtained using the hybrid DARCES–ICP algorithm, could potentially result in an MSE value that is lower than that obtained using the hybrid DARCES–ICP algorithm. The coefficients of the functional approximation $(\lambda_1, \lambda_2, \lambda_3)$ are computed as follows:

$$\frac{\lambda_1}{|\Delta(\epsilon^2)|} = \frac{\lambda_2}{|\Delta(\psi^{-1})|} = \frac{\lambda_3}{|\Delta(\bar{A})|} \quad \text{and} \\ \sum_{i=1}^{3}(\lambda_i) = 1, \tag{4.43}$$

where $\Delta(x)$ denotes the normalized absolute difference (i.e., the difference of the maximum and minimum values, divided by the maximum value) of the variable x over the range of perturbations.

4.11 Experimental Results

In this section, we first discuss the experimental results of various surface matching algorithms on a typical phantom dataset (i.e., CT images of a phantom mandible subject to simulated craniofacial trauma) and a typical real patient dataset (i.e., CT images of a human mandible that has experienced real craniofacial trauma). Next, we demonstrate the effectiveness of the composite reconstruction scheme which incorporates shape symmetry, biomechanical stability, and angular perturbation within a single reconstruction metric by showing experimental results on a phantom CT dataset.

Table 4.3 compares the reconstruction accuracy of the ICP, the DARCES, and the hybrid DARCES–ICP algorithms for a typical phantom dataset and a typical real patient dataset. In both the cases, the hybrid DARCES–ICP algorithm clearly outperforms the individual ICP and DARCES algorithms in terms of reconstruction accuracy. In addition, the convergence of the hybrid DARCES–ICP algorithm is achieved within 3–4 iterations in comparison to 6–8 iterations of the original

Table 4.3 MSE values resulting from the DARCES, ICP and hybrid DARCES–ICP algorithms

Datasets	MSE–DAR. (mm^2)	MSE–ICP (mm^2)	MSE–Hyb. DAR.–ICP (mm^2)
Phantom	0.33	0.91	0.25
Real	4.62	2.07	1.24

Table 4.4 MSE values resulting from the hybrid DARCES–ICP algorithm using three different synergism strategies

Level of Synergism	MSE for hybrid DARCES–ICP (mm^2)
Synergism-1	2.07
Synergism-2	1.65
Synergism-3	1.24

Table 4.5 MSE values resulting from the hybrid DARCES–ICP algorithm with various reward–penalty schemes

Scheme	Penalty Coeff. (λ)	MSE (mm^2)
hybrid DARCES–ICP	–	0.251
hybrid DARCES–ICP + Fuzzy Set based	1.0	0.254
hybrid DARCES–ICP + Fuzzy Set based	0.5	0.235
hybrid DARCES–ICP + Fuzzy Set based	0.1	0.248
hybrid DARCES–ICP + Curvature based	1.0	0.252
hybrid DARCES–ICP + Curvature based	0.5	0.247
hybrid DARCES–ICP + Curvature based	0.1	0.234

ICP algorithm. However, in the case where each fracture surface dataset consists of only the interest points (essentially points of high curvature), both the DARCES and the ICP algorithms take only a few seconds more than the hybrid DARCES–ICP algorithm for completion. For example, in the case of real patient CT data, all the three algorithms finished their execution within well less than a minute on a 1.73-GHz Intel Pentium-M© processor. Thus, it can be inferred that although the hybrid DARCES–ICP algorithm yields a lower surface matching error (MSE), its computational benefit (in terms of execution time) over the ICP algorithm used in isolation is perceivable only in cases where the input datasets to the ICP algorithm are very dense. In dense datasets, the DARCES component of the hybrid DARCES–ICP algorithm can be used to greatly prune substantially the sample dataset by virtue of outlier removal. Consequently, the ICP component of the hybrid DARCES–ICP algorithm runs on a considerably sparser sample dataset, resulting in a perceivably lower computation time.

Table 4.4 shows the impact of exploiting the various levels of synergism between the ICP and DARCES algorithms (discussed in Sect. 4.5.3) on the MSE. It is interesting to note that not all the ways of exploiting synergism between the DARCES and ICP algorithms are equally effective. The subset of the sample dataset that is properly aligned by the DARCES algorithm consists of the original sample dataset with potential outliers removed. When the ICP algorithm is run on this filtered dataset, with the initial transformation estimate as the output of the DARCES algorithm (i.e., *Synergism 3*), the lowest overall MSE is achieved.

Table 4.5 demonstrates the impact of modeling the irregularities of a typical fracture surface. Note that the modeling of these irregularities is necessary but not sufficient to guarantee a better reconstruction. The tuning of the penalty coefficient λ

plays an important role in the performance of the scheme. This fact is evident from Table 4.5, where only certain values of the penalty coefficient are observed to yield an MSE value lower than that resulting from the hybrid DARCES–ICP algorithm. Since the hybrid DARCES–ICP algorithm generates an MSE value which is very close to the global minimum for a given pair of opposing fracture surfaces, an appropriate choice of the penalty coefficient would guide the algorithm toward the global minimum (resulting in further decrease of the observed MSE value), whereas an inappropriate choice would guide the algorithm away from the global minimum (resulting in an increase in the observed MSE value).

We have experimentally verified the improvement in the surface registration error using the hybrid Geometric–ICP algorithm in place of the conventional ICP algorithm. As mentioned earlier, in the Geometric–ICP algorithm, the bounding box for a fracture surface is modeled as a cycle graph of order four. Thus, there are a total of eight possible automorphs to be considered. Let the vertices of the bounding box B_1 be denoted by $M - N - O - P$, and those of B_2 by $P - Q - R - S$. Then the members of the automorphism group of B_2 are given by

1. $P - Q - R - S$, $S - P - Q - R$, $R - S - P - Q$, $Q - R - S - P$ (4 rotational automorphs).
2. $Q - P - S - R$, $P - S - R - Q$, $S - R - Q - P$, $R - Q - P - S$ (4 reflectional automorphs).

The top 50%, i.e., four out of eight, automorphs are selected based on the value of the dissimilarity function $\Gamma(B_1, AB_{2,l})$ (see Table 4.6 and (4.25)). The best four candidate transformations $\phi_1, \dots, \phi_4$ are then estimated from B_1 and the best four automorphs and applied to the bone fragment frg_1 resulting in the four reconstructed mandibles $M_1, \dots, M_4$.

Figure 4.5 shows the reference contour Co_{ref} in the first row and the contours of the four registered mandibles $Co_1, \dots, Co_4$ (obtained using the corresponding transformations $\phi_1, \dots, \phi_4$) in the second and third rows. Table 4.7 shows the CHD values obtained using (4.26), from which the best matching contour Co^* ($= Co_2$ in the current example) and the corresponding transformation ϕ^* ($= \phi_2$ in the current example) are estimated. Figure 4.5 clearly demonstrates how multiple competing opposable fracture surfaces and thereby multiple candidate solutions for the reconstructed mandible are generated and how the best (coarse) solution, denoted by the corresponding rigid body transformation ϕ^*, is obtained. As described earlier, the algorithm leading to the best coarse solution is termed as the Geometric algorithm since the resulting solution is based on satisfaction of certain predefined relational geometric constraints, i.e., *type-1* constraints.

Table 4.8 and Fig. 4.6 respectively describe, quantitatively and qualitatively, the performance of various reconstruction algorithms on a real (human) craniofacial fracture. It is interesting to observe that both, the DARCES algorithm and the Geometric algorithm, yield similar reconstruction accuracy. The ICP algorithm, by itself, performed better than either the DARCES algorithm or the Geometric algorithm. The synergism between the DARCES algorithm and the ICP algorithm and the synergism between the Geometric algorithm and the ICP algorithm are observed

Table 4.6 Dissimilarity function values for competing automorphs

Automorph Rank	Dissimilarity Function Value
1	52.20
2	57.30
3	61.37
4	66.51

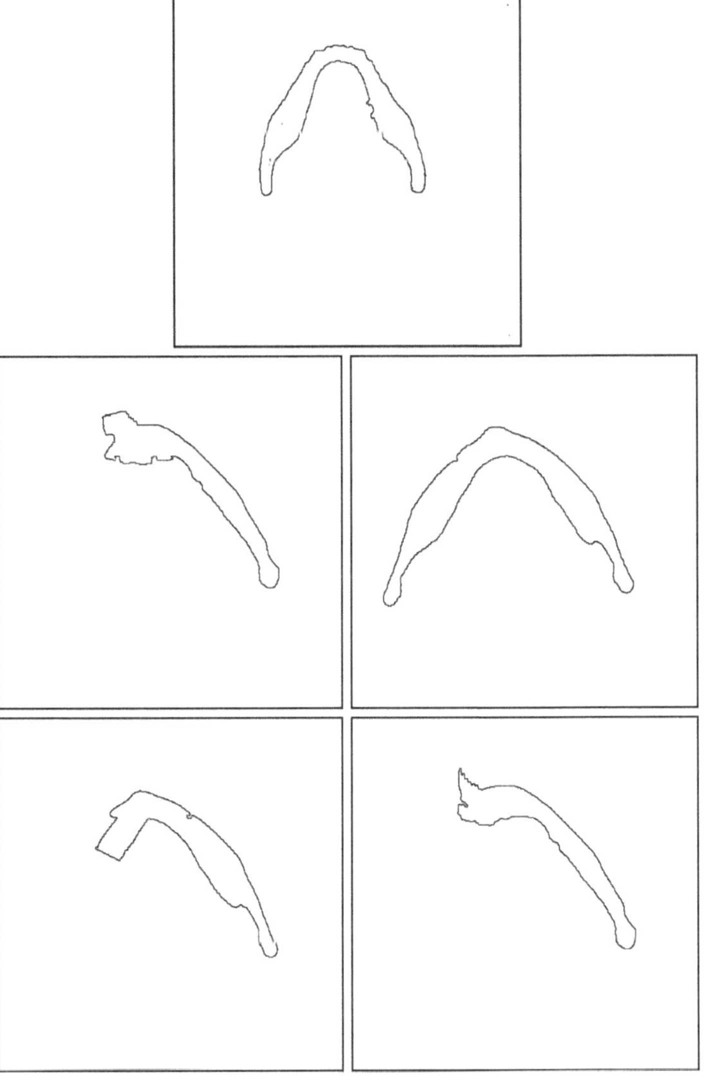

Fig. 4.5 Reference contour in the *first row*. Four differently registered contours in the *second* and *third rows*

Table 4.7 CHD values for competing contours

Contour from Fig. 4.5	Rank	CHD Value
Co_1	1	111.22
Co_2	2	2.24
Co_3	3	52.43
Co_4	4	149.97

Table 4.8 MSE for five different reconstruction algorithms for a typical dataset

Reconstruction Algorithm	MSE (mm^2)
DARCES	4.62
ICP	2.07
hybrid DARCES–ICP	1.24
Geometric	4.57
hybrid Geometric–ICP	1.96

to further improve the reconstruction accuracy. Since the best reconstruction accuracy is obtained using the hybrid DARCES–ICP algorithm, the volume rendering of a fractured mandible (of a real patient) and its reconstructed version using the hybrid DARCES–ICP algorithm is illustrated in Fig. 4.7. In Fig. 4.8, the slice-wise reconstruction results for a phantom mandible using the DARCES algorithm, the ICP algorithm, and the hybrid DARCES–ICP algorithm are presented. A visual comparison of the projections of a 3D intact (i.e., prior to fracture) phantom mandible and a 3D reconstructed phantom mandible along the X, Y, and Z axes is shown in Fig. 4.9.

Table 4.9 shows typical values for the coefficient of symmetry for the three different candidate planes in the unperturbed state. The variations of the (a) mean squared error (ϵ^2), (b) inverse coefficient of symmetry for the plane of bilateral symmetry (ψ^{-1}), (c) average surface area ($\bar{A}$), and (d) normalized composite reconstruction metric (CRM) as a function of angular perturbations along each of the three major axes are graphically portrayed in Figs. 4.10, 4.11, 4.12, and 4.13, respectively. The values of the coefficients λ_1, λ_2, and λ_3 of ϵ^2, ψ^{-1}, and $\bar{A}$, respectively (4.41) are shown in Table 4.10. With the incorporation of very small angular perturbations, it is possible to attain a reconstruction state, which not only yields better results in terms of the average surface area and shape symmetry, but also reduces the local MSE. This is clearly demonstrated in Table 4.11, where the first and second rows show the values of the MSE, inverse shape symmetry, and average surface area for the unperturbed configuration (i.e., the reconstruction generated by the hybrid DARCES–ICP algorithm) and the optimal configuration (resulting from a perturbation of $-0.4°$ about the X-axis, resulting in the minimum normalized CRM value), respectively. These results show the effectiveness of the incorporation of the bilateral symmetry and the biomechanical stability in the proposed virtual reconstruction scheme.

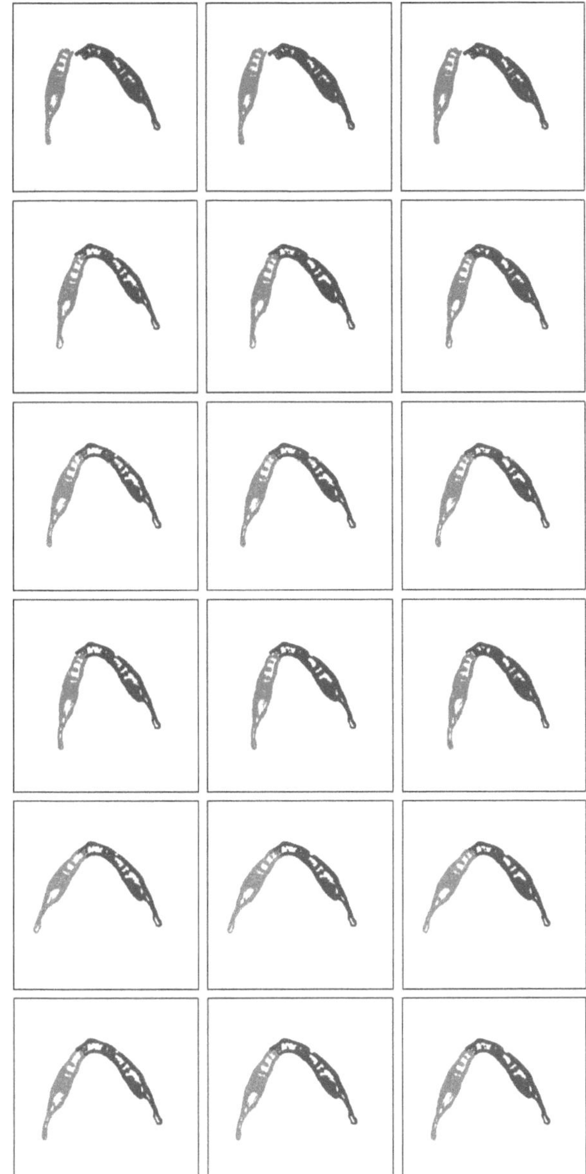

Fig. 4.6 CT image slices of a fractured human mandible (*first row*). Slice-wise reconstruction results using the DARCES algorithm (*second row*), ICP algorithm (*third row*), hybrid DARCES–ICP algorithm (*fourth row*), Geometric algorithm (*fifth row*), hybrid Geometric–ICP algorithm (*sixth row*)

4.12 Conclusion and Future Work

This chapter addressed various aspects of 3D virtual craniofacial reconstruction from CT images exhibiting single fractures. A single 3D CT image stack was treated as a sequence of 2D images for the purpose of feature extraction and displaying the registered images. We tackled the problem of 3D mandibular reconstruction as a single problem of 3D registration using a 3D CT image stack instead of a series of

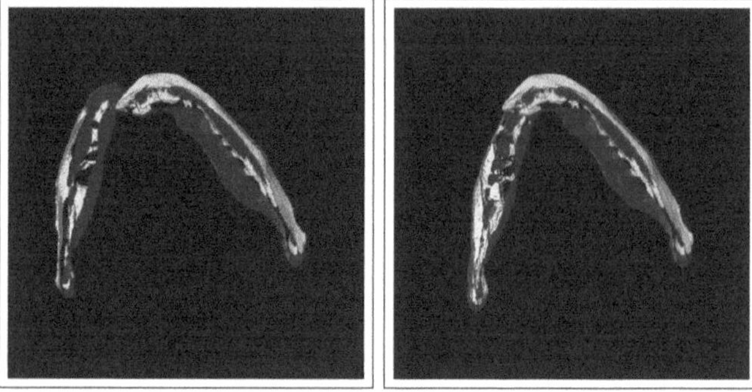

Fig. 4.7 Volume rendering of the fractured mandible and the reconstructed mandible (using the hybrid DARCES–ICP algorithm)

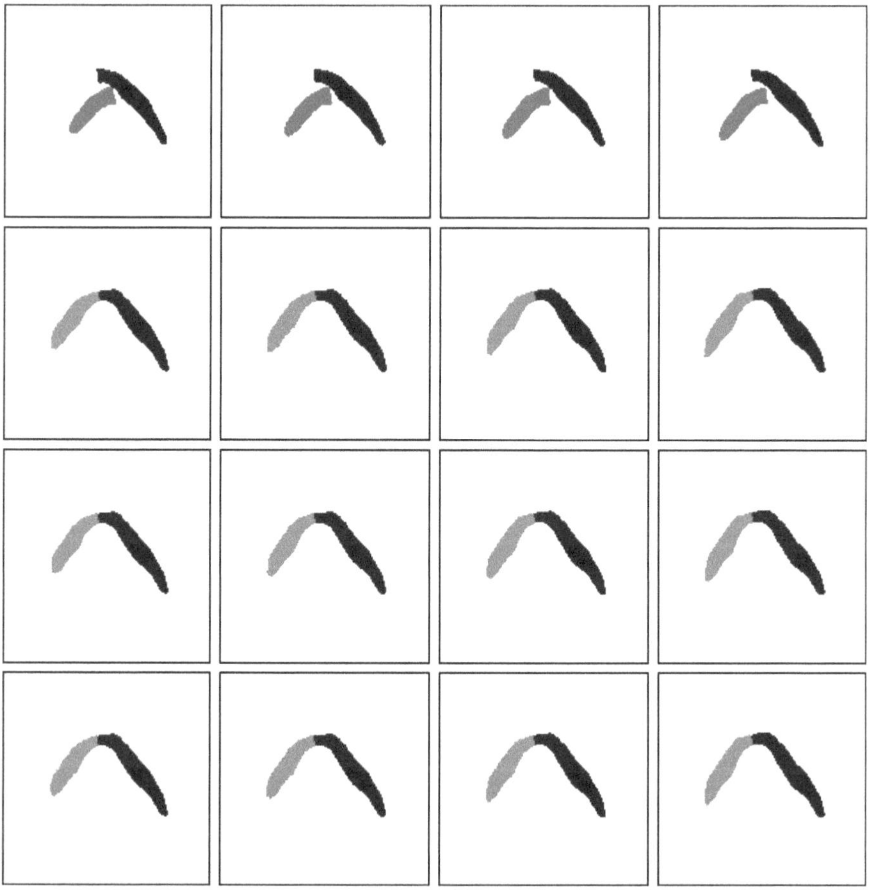

Fig. 4.8 The *first row* depicts CT image slices from a fractured phantom mandible subject to simulated craniofacial trauma. The *second*, *third*, and *fourth rows* depict the CT image slices from the reconstructed mandible resulting from the DARCES algorithm, ICP algorithm, and hybrid DARCES–ICP algorithm, respectively

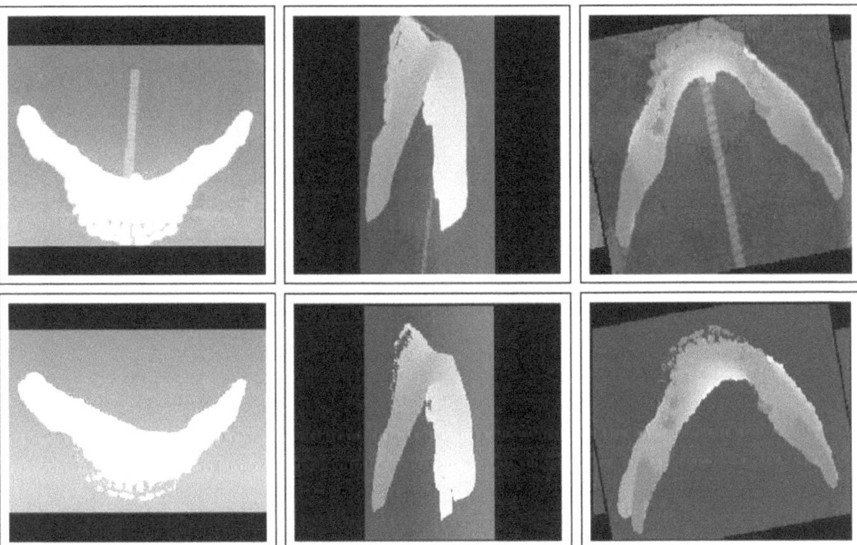

Fig. 4.9 Comparison of the original phantom mandible (prior to fracture) and the reconstructed phantom mandible (post fracture). The *top row* represents the original mandible, and the *bottom row* is the reconstructed mandible obtained using hybrid DARCES–ICP algorithm. The *first*, *second*, and *third columns* represent the 3D projections along the X, Y, and Z axes, respectively

Table 4.9 Plane of symmetry and coefficient of symmetry for a phantom dataset in an unperturbed state

Coeff. of Sym.	Eqn. of the Candidate Planes of Symm.	Comments
0.79	$0.98x - 0.16y + 0.12z = 65.42$	Plane of Bilateral Symm.
0.27	$-0.20x + 0.87y - 0.45z = 58.78$	–
0.35	$-0.03x + 0.47y + 0.88z = 50.95$	–

slice-wise 2D registration problems. Two different types of algorithms, namely the ICP algorithm and the DARCES algorithm, were first applied individually and then in a cascaded manner for accurate surface matching. The combination of these two algorithms, termed as the hybrid DARCES–ICP algorithm, resulted in an improved mean squared surface matching error (MSE) and a significant reduction in the execution time when compared to the ICP algorithm used in isolation. The irregularities on the fracture surfaces were modeled using the theory of mean and Gaussian curvatures from differential surface geometry and the theory of fuzzy sets. The MSE resulting from the DARCES–ICP algorithm was further reduced by incorporating the fracture surface irregularity information within the reconstruction paradigm by means of two reward–penalty schemes. Note that all the above algorithms exploited the point set representation of the fracture surfaces, i.e., the algorithms satisfied *type-0* constraints.

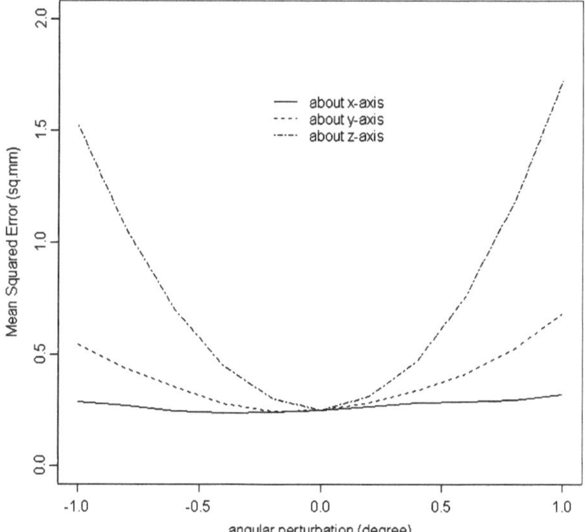

Fig. 4.10 Variation in the MSE (ϵ^2) with angular perturbation along all the three major axes

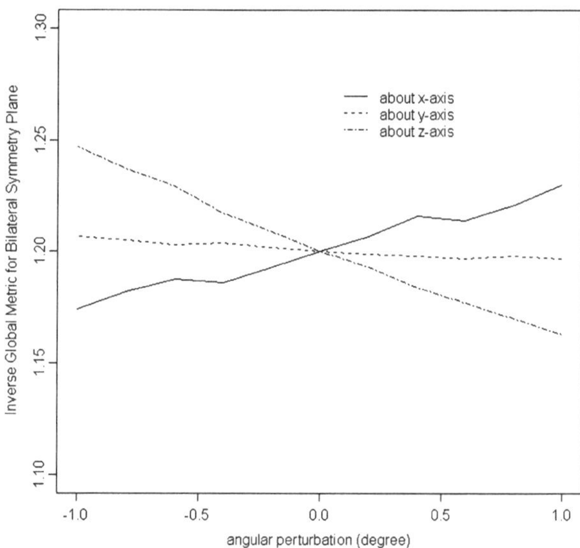

Fig. 4.11 Variation in the inverse coefficient of symmetry (ψ^{-1}) with angular perturbation along all the three major axes

In an alternative formulation, the fracture surface was described as a solid object with a well-defined bounding box. This motivated the design of the Geometric algorithm and hybrid Geometric–ICP algorithm based on satisfaction of certain predefined relational geometric constraints termed as *type-1* constraints. The hybrid DARCES–ICP algorithm was seen to benefit mainly from outlier rejection in the fracture surface datasets. The hybrid Geometric–ICP algorithm, on the other hand, took advantage of satisfying the predefined relational geometric constraints. Next, we focused on preservation of the bilateral symmetry and biomechanical stability

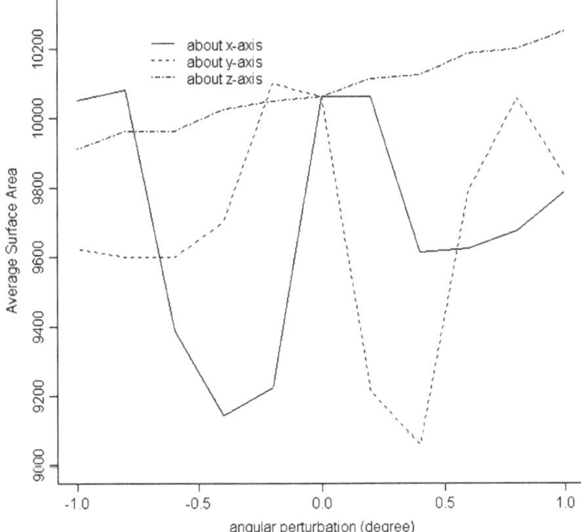

Fig. 4.12 Variation in the average surface area ($\bar{A}$) with angular perturbation along all the three major axes

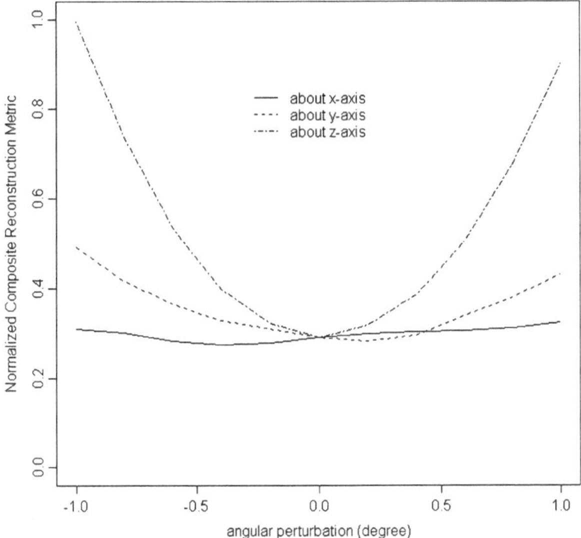

Fig. 4.13 Variation in the Normalized *CRM* with angular perturbation along all the three major axes

of the reconstructed human mandible in addition to ensuring accurate local surface matching. Since the human mandible is known to exhibit bilateral symmetry, the plane of bilateral symmetry was computed using a normalized cross-correlation procedure. Minimization of surface area was shown to be mathematically equivalent to minimization of surface energy and was used as a measure of biomechanical stability. The plane of bilateral symmetry and average surface area were estimated for the reconstructed mandible resulting from the hybrid DARCES–ICP algorithm. A composite reconstruction metric (*CRM*), formulated as a linear combination of the mean squared surface matching error, the inverse of a global shape symmetry

Table 4.10 Coefficients of the *CRM* terms for a phantom dataset

λ_1 (Coeff. of ϵ^2)	λ_2 (Coeff. of ψ^{-1})	λ_3 (Coeff. of $\bar{A}$)
0.82	0.06	0.11

Table 4.11 Comparison of performance measures for a phantom dataset in the unperturbed and optimal states

State	ϵ^2	ψ^{-1}	$\bar{A}$	Ω
Optimal $(x, -0.4^0)$	0.138	0.952	0.892	0.275
Unperturbed $(-, -)$	0.148	0.964	0.982	0.293

measure, and the mandibular surface area, was subsequently introduced as a performance measure for the reconstruction process. A local search based on an angular perturbation scheme, in this phase, was shown to result in a solution that minimizes not only the MSE but also the composite reconstruction metric.

As a part of future research, we plan to build anatomical models of the reconstructed mandible. These models could be used to generate useful feedback on the virtual reconstruction process. For example, one could use the feedback to automatically fine tune the coefficients of the three different factors in the composite reconstruction metric to ensure a more anatomically meaningful reconstruction. We envisage the possible use of a robotic arm to perform the surgery under the supervision of an experienced surgeon. The robotic arm could use the 3D rigid body transformation, resulting from one of the various reconstruction algorithms, to put the fractured fragments into registration. Another direction for future work, as mentioned earlier, would be the replacement of the bounding box of a fracture surface by its convex hull in the Geometric and Geometric–ICP algorithms. Finally, it would be interesting to attempt and evaluate further combinations of the surface matching algorithms such as incorporating the fracture surface irregularity information within the hybrid Geometric–ICP algorithm and formulation of a hybrid DARCES–Geometric–ICP algorithm.

Chapter 5
Virtual Multiple-Fracture Mandibular Reconstruction

5.1 Motivation

From a surgical perspective, the craniofacial reconstruction problem assumes even greater complexity when faced with multiple fractures since the operating surgeon has to identify the opposable fracture surfaces before physically registering them. Very often, the cost of surgery becomes prohibitive with the increased operative time necessary to complete the entire reconstruction process [3]. Moreover, the increased operative time also poses increased operative trauma and an increased risk of postoperative complications to the patient.

The reconstruction problem, in the case of multiple fractures, falls essentially within the category of automated jigsaw puzzle solving. Automated jigsaw puzzle solving is of general interest in a variety of domains ranging from archeology to forensics that often deal with problems related to automated reconstruction or assembly. The input to our specific problem of automated craniofacial reconstruction is a Computed Tomography (CT) scan of a human mandible that exhibits multiple fractures. After performing simple image processing operations on the CT images, the broken bone fragments are separated from the soft tissue. The fracture surfaces on the broken bone fragments are manually highlighted by the surgeon. It is for this reason that we deem our multiple-fracture reconstruction scheme to be semi-automated instead of one that is fully automated.

A novel two-step scheme based on graph matching is proposed as a solution to the multiple-fracture registration problem. In the first step, the opposable fracture surfaces are identified using the Maximum Weight Graph Matching (MWGM) algorithm for a weighted graph. The fracture surfaces are modeled as vertices of a weighted graph. The edge weights in the graph are chosen as a linear combination of (a) the inverse Hausdorff distance and (b) an appropriately formulated function of contour curvature. In the second step, the opposable fracture surface pairs, identified in the first step, are registered using the Iterative Closest Point (ICP) algorithm. The pointwise surface correspondence between fracture surface pairs during each iteration of the ICP algorithm is determined using the Maximum Cardinality Minimum Weight (MCMW) bipartite graph matching algorithm. The reconstruction process

A.S. Chowdhury, S.M. Bhandarkar, *Computer Vision-Guided Virtual Craniofacial Surgery*, Advances in Computer Vision and Pattern Recognition,
DOI 10.1007/978-0-85729-296-4_5,

in the second step is continuously monitored using global shape constraints derived from a volumetric matching procedure that is guided by the computation of the Tanimoto Coefficient.

5.2 Chapter Organization

The remainder of the chapter is organized into eight different sections. Section 5.3 describes the existing related work and highlights our contribution. Section 5.4 describes the various image processing procedures necessary to obtain data from the segmented fracture surfaces. The material in this section is similar to that in Sect. 4.4 and hence not discussed in great detail. Section 5.5 details the formulation of the score matrix needed as input to the MWGM algorithm. This section contains three subsections. In Sect. 5.5.1, we model mathematically the spatial proximity of the fracture surfaces. In Sect. 5.5.2, we model mathematically the fracture surface characteristics. In Sect. 5.5.3, we discuss the generation of the elements of the score matrix. Next, in Sect. 5.6, we describe how the juxtaposable fracture surface pairs are identified. This section has two separate subsections. In Sect. 5.6.1, we prove the combinatorial nature of the problem in terms of the number of reconstruction possibilities. In Sect. 5.6.2, we illustrate how the MWGM algorithm actually identifies the opposable fracture surface pairs. Section 5.7 describes the pairwise registration of the fracture surfaces using the ICP algorithm. Once again, the correspondence problem within the ICP algorithm is solved using the MCMW bipartite graph matching algorithm. Note that any of the other registration algorithms discussed in the previous chapter, namely, the DARCES, the hybrid DARCES–ICP, the Geometric, and the hybrid Geometric–ICP algorithms could also be employed for this purpose. Since the material in this section is essentially the same as that presented in Sect. 4.5.1, we choose to skip the details. Section 5.8 details the shape monitoring procedure based on the computation of the Tanimoto coefficient. In Sect. 5.9, we present the experimental results and their analyses. Finally, the chapter is concluded in Sect. 5.10 with directions for future research.

5.3 Related Work and Our Contribution

The multiple-fracture craniofacial reconstruction problem, in a broader sense, can be viewed as a combinatorial pattern matching problem that is similar to automated jigsaw puzzle solving. We first discuss various existing approaches for solving the two-dimensional (2D) and three-dimensional (3D) jigsaw puzzle problem. The significance of multiple mandibular and craniofacial fractures in the surgical literature is presented next. The section is concluded by highlighting our contribution in the context of the multiple-fracture reconstruction problem.

Since there exist several published works in the research literature on automated jigsaw puzzle solving, we restrict ourselves to the discussion of a few representative works. The research on automated jigsaw puzzle solving by means of a computer, using images as input, was initiated almost two decades ago with the work of Wolfson et al. [87]. In their seminal paper, they model the 2D jigsaw puzzle solving problem as the well-known Traveling Salesperson Problem (TSP). Webster et al. [88] identify critical isthmus points as robust global features for matching the pieces of a 2D jigsaw puzzle. The critical isthmus points are extracted using a medial axis transformation. Leitato and Stolfi [89] use multiscale filtering and an initial matching followed by refinement and pruning of the search space with incremental dynamic programming to solve the 2D jigsaw puzzle problem. Yao and Shao [90] present an algorithm which combines shape and image matching with a cyclic "growth" process that tries to place the 2D jigsaw puzzle pieces in their correct positions. Goldberg et al. [91], on the other hand, address the problem of 2D jigsaw puzzle reconstruction using a global relaxation approach after detection of fiducial points (i.e., robust canonical locations) on the 2D jigsaw puzzle pieces.

The previously mentioned works have dealt with 2D jigsaw puzzle solving, whereas more recent research has focused on jigsaw puzzle solving in three dimensions. Makridis and Papamarkos [92] propose a new technique for 3D jigsaw puzzle solving which employs both geometrical and color features for matching the jigsaw puzzle pieces. Barequet and Sharir [93] present improved 3D geometric hashing techniques for partial surface and volume matching for solving 3D jigsaw puzzles. Ucoluk and Toroslu [94] model the 3D jigsaw puzzle solving problem as one of matching two 3D space curves. Papaioannou et al. [95] formulate a novel matching error metric for solving the 3D reconstruction problem via matching of individual parts using a 3D shape signature. Huang et al. [96] use integral invariants in the process of matching geometrically the fragments of 3D objects.

Some other important instances of the 3D jigsaw puzzle solving problem include the archaeological fragment assembly problem by Kampel and Sablantig [97]. The 3D earthenware assembly problem presented by Willis and Cooper [98] can also be regarded as an instance of 3D jigsaw puzzle solving. In their formulation of the 3D earthenware assembly problem, Willis and Cooper [98] use axially symmetric shape descriptors for the broken fragments in conjunction with a Bayesian reconstruction procedure. Note that 3D jigsaw puzzle solving is an example of a computationally intractable NP-hard problem in the area of computer vision and pattern recognition. Some other problems in the same category include planar shape prototype generation as discussed by Chen et al. [99], minimum distance problems with convex or concave bodies as described by Carreto and Nihan [100] and the multimode test sequencing problem discussed by Ruan et al. [101].

In an article by Ogundare et al. [2], it was shown that 52% of the patients, studied in a typical urban-level trauma center, suffered from multiple mandibular fractures. In a study conducted by Boole et al. [102], about 30% of the army soldiers who experienced craniofacial trauma while on active duty were seen to suffer from two or more mandibular fractures. Clauser et al. [103] discuss the prevalence of severe midface fractures as a result of vehicular accidents, which could lead to surgical

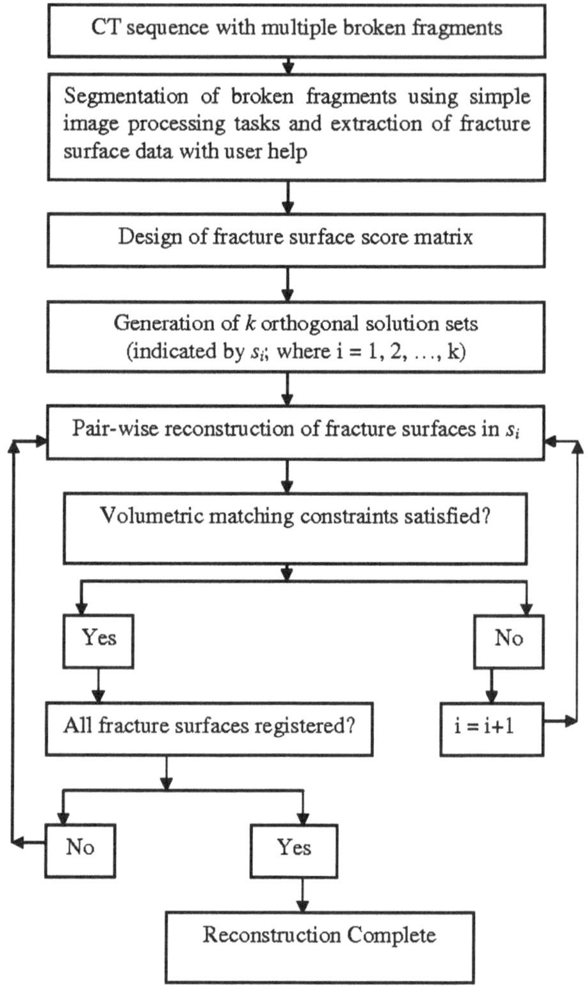

Fig. 5.1 Flowchart for virtual multiple-fracture reconstruction

procedures involving high clinical complexity. It is interesting to note that in their work on multiple craniofacial injuries, Schettler et al. [104] suggest that the surgical reconstruction technique used in the case of craniofacial trauma is often tantamount to solving a jigsaw puzzle.

Graph matching algorithms have been frequently employed to solve various problems in computer vision, see, e.g., the work by Chen et al. [105]. Here, we use general graph matching and bipartite graph matching algorithms in novel ways at different stages of the multiple-fracture reconstruction procedure [106]. A flowchart of the proposed multiple-fracture reconstruction scheme is shown in Fig. 5.1 [107]. As shown in Fig. 5.1, the reconstruction process is complete only after all the fracture surface pairs in a solution set s_i, derived from the MWGM algorithm, are registered in a manner that satisfies the volumetric matching constraints. The primary contribution of the paper lies in proposing the MWGM algorithm for identification of opposable fracture surface pairs in a CT scan of a patient who has suffered severe craniofacial trauma. To the best of our knowledge, no work has been reported thus far which uses a graph matching-based approach for assembling a 3D jigsaw puzzle. A novel score matrix formulation which assists the graph matching algorithm in generating an optimal solution is presented. As mentioned earlier, the score matrix elements reflect the property of spatial proximity and the desirable surface characteristics between two opposable fracture surfaces. The second important contribution lies in the design of the MCMW algorithm for establishing a correspondence between two fracture surfaces while registering them using the ICP algorithm. Finally, the monitoring of the reconstruction process at each step using volumetric constraints also deserves special mention.

5.4 Image Processing

The input to the multiple-fracture mandibular reconstruction procedure is a sequence of 2D grayscale CT images of a human mandible exhibiting multiple fractures. Figure 5.2 shows three consecutive CT slices of such an image sequence. The image processing tasks of thresholding and connected component labeling, described in the previous chapter, are undertaken to segment the broken bone fragments from the surrounding tissue.

The result of the simple thresholding is shown in Fig. 5.3, where the pixels denoting the broken fragments are represented by the highest intensity value, and the remaining pixels by the lowest intensity value. A 2D Connected Component Labeling (CCL) procedure is used on the binary image. The results of the 2D CCL procedure are propagated across the CT image slices, resulting in a 3D CCL algorithm. A 3D component (a fractured jaw bone in this case) is identified by computing the area of overlap of the corresponding 2D components in successive CT image slices.

The result of the CCL procedure is shown in Fig. 5.4, where the six broken fragments are represented by six different grayscale values, and the background pixels are assigned the highest intensity value for better visualization. In the current implementation, the fracture surfaces on the broken bone fragments are manually iden-

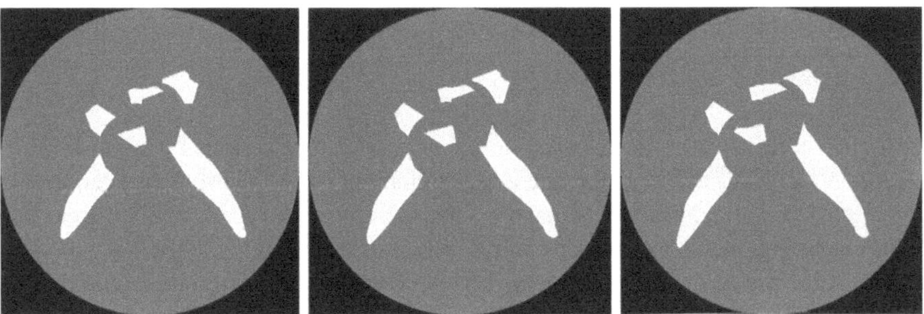

Fig. 5.2 Input CT image sequence of a phantom mandible exhibiting multiple fractures (3 consecutive slices shown)

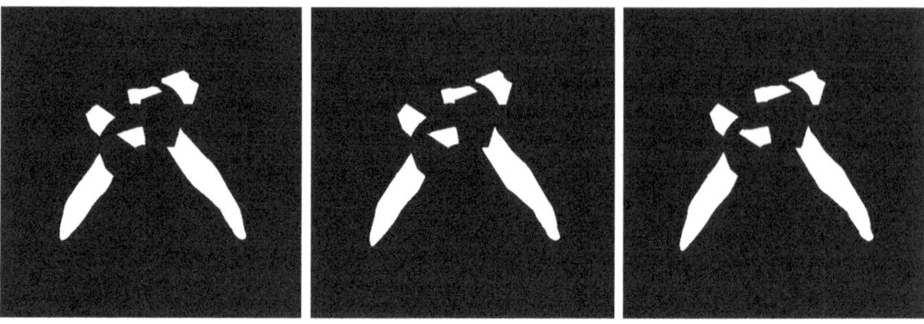

Fig. 5.3 Result of simple thresholding (on the slices in Fig. 5.2)

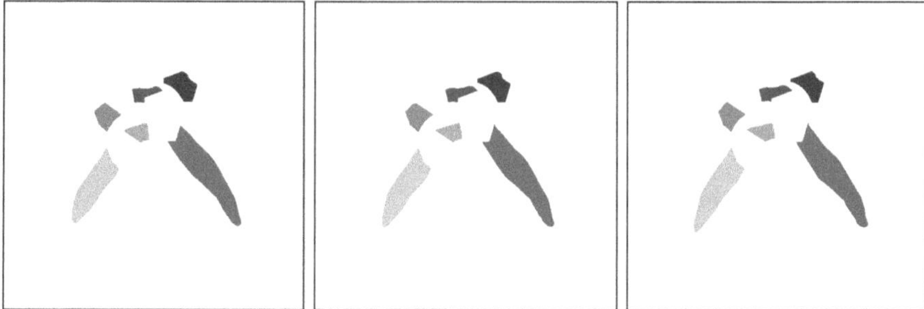

Fig. 5.4 Result of connected component labeling (on the slices in Fig. 5.2)

tified by the surgeon. The task of interactive contour data extraction is performed next on each of the binary image slices. The contour points, obtained from the individual binary image slices, are collated to generate the 3D surface point dataset. A 3D surface point dataset is thus generated for each fracture surface. The fracture surface data is used as input for solving the combinatorial pattern matching problem and generating the 3D transformation for surface registration. The 3D transformation thus obtained is then applied to the appropriate bone fragments for the purpose of virtual reconstruction.

5.5 Design of a Score Matrix

A score matrix is formulated based on the appearance of various mandibular fragments in the input CT image sequence. An element of the score matrix represents the degree of compatibility between the corresponding pair of fracture surfaces. The mandibular fragments are classified as *terminal* or *nonterminal*, based on the presence or absence of condyles, respectively. A condyle is an extremity of the human mandible that exhibits pronounced sphericity. This prior rudimentary classification of the bone fragments to be assembled bears resemblance to the schemes proposed by Wolfson et al. [87] and Goldberg et al. [91] in the context of automated jigsaw

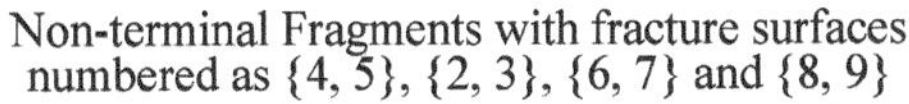

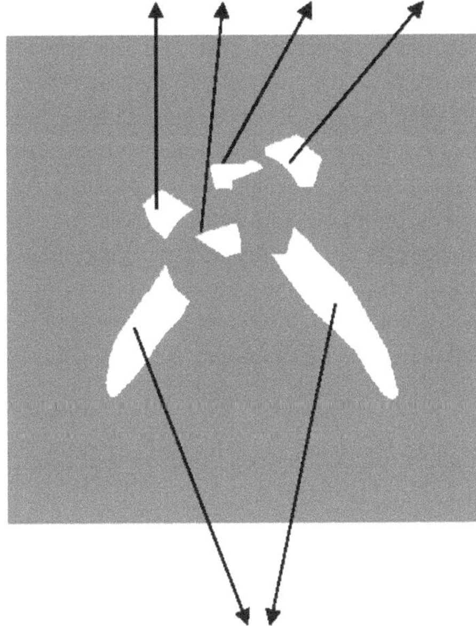

Fig. 5.5 A single 2D slice showing the terminal and nonterminal fragments with the associated fracture contours

puzzle solving. Both Wolfson et al. and Goldberg et al. assemble separately the *border* and *interior* frame pieces of a jigsaw puzzle. In fact, Goldberg et al. further classify the border pieces as indents, outdents, and flat sides. A terminal fragment, in our case, is analogous to a border piece of a jigsaw puzzle, whereas a nonterminal fragment is analogous to an interior piece of a jigsaw puzzle. A terminal fragment is often found to contain a single fracture surface. By contrast, a nonterminal fragment often exhibits two fracture surfaces (see Fig. 5.5).

In the present work, the mathematical formulation, experiments, and subsequent mathematical analysis of the experimental results are based on the assumption that a terminal fragment has one fracture surface and a nonterminal fragment has two fracture surfaces. However, the proposed scheme is flexible enough to handle any number of fracture surfaces for a given fragment. Each fracture surface is represented by a collection of 3D data points obtained by extracting and collating the corresponding fracture contour points in the individual 2D CT image slices. In the case of 2D jigsaw puzzle solving, the score matrix formulation is based typically on curve matching, where the matrix elements denote the compatibility between potentially opposable edge points [108, 109]. In our case, we need to estimate the matching score between the 3D fracture surfaces extracted from the CT image slices. A high matching score is assigned to a pair of fracture surfaces if (a) they are determined to be spatially proximal and (b) they are determined to exhibit complementary (opposable) fracture surface characteristics. We have used both of these factors in determining the matching score for the proposed score matrix formulation.

5.5.1 Modeling Spatial Proximity

The various fracture surfaces under consideration possess a varying number of data points. The formulation of a distance measure, i.e., a measure of spatial separation, between any surface pair requires the establishment of correspondence between the data points on the two surfaces. Given the high dimensionality of the score matrix, determined by the number of possible fracture surface pairs for which the above correspondence has to be established a priori, the task of determining a distance measure is computationally very expensive. Therefore, we use the Hausdorff distance, which does not need prior determination of correspondence between the two data point sets to yield a measure of spatial separation between them. The Hausdorff distance $H(A, B)$ between two datasets A and B is given by [74]

$$H(A, B) = \max\big(h(A, B), h(B, A)\big), \tag{5.1}$$

where $h(A, B)$ denotes the *directed* Hausdorff distance between the two datasets A and B and is defined as

$$h(A, B) = \max_{a\in A} \min_{b\in B} \|a - b\|. \tag{5.2}$$

Here $\|a - b\|$ represents the Euclidean distance between the points a and b. Note that each of the variables a and b, in our case, denotes a 3D data point in the fracture surface data set A and B, respectively. The computation of the Hausdorff distance can be performed directly in $O(mn)$ time, i.e., quadratic polynomial time, where m and n denote the cardinalities of the two fracture surface data sets under consideration.

5.5.2 Modeling Surface Characteristics

There are well-known measures for characterizing 3D surfaces described in the computer vision literature of which the *Gaussian* and *mean* curvatures are the most prominent [67]. Each fracture surface in the present scenario is viewed as a collection of several fracture contours. It is to be noted that the determination of the Gaussian and mean curvatures is computationally more intensive and more sensitive to noise compared to the determination of contour curvature. The choice of contour curvature as a measure of surface irregularity is further justified by the fact that it also possesses the properties of rotational and translational invariance [110]. The *contour curvature* for a point (x, y) in a given CT image slice (i.e., for a specific value of z) is given by [110]

$$c(x, y) = \big(d^2y/dx^2\big)/\big(1 + (dy/dx)^2\big)^{3/2}. \tag{5.3}$$

We formulate a function which captures the compatibility between two fracture surfaces using contour curvature. The function $FS(A, B)$ for a pair of surfaces A, B is defined as the sum of the scores $fs(a, b)$ for each possible point pair, one point from each of the surfaces. If the two points under consideration have the same signs for their contour curvatures, then they cause the overall surface matching score to increase; otherwise they cause it to decrease. Thus, we can write

$$FS(A, B) = \sum_{a \in A} \sum_{b \in B} fs(a, b). \tag{5.4}$$

Intuitively, the score $fs(a, b)$ between any pair of points a and b is high if (a) the slice-wise locations of the two points are spatially proximal, (b) the relative positions of the two points in their respective slices are proximal (where the relative position of a fracture point in a slice is measured with respect to the end points, in the same slice, of the fracture contour on which the fracture point lies), and (c) the curvature values of the two points are close. The score will be low if any of the above criteria is not satisfied. Thus, we can quantitatively express $fs(a, b)$ as the product of the above three factors and a sign function as follows:

$$fs(a, b) = S(a, b)E(a, b)C(a, b)sg(c_a c_b), \tag{5.5}$$

where

$$\begin{aligned}
S(a, b) &= 2/\big(1 + \exp\big(|s_a - s_b|\big)\big), \\
E(a, b) &= 2/\big(1 + \exp\big(|e_a - e_b|\big)\big), \\
C(a, b) &= 2/\big(1 + \exp\big(|c_a - c_b|\big)\big), \\
sg(c_a c_b) &= \begin{cases} +1 & \text{if } c_a c_b > 0, \\ -1 & \text{if } c_a c_b < 0. \end{cases}
\end{aligned} \tag{5.6}$$

Here $S(a, b)$, $E(a, b)$, and $C(a, b)$ respectively denote the slice-wise location-based score, relative position within the slice-based score, and the curvature value-based score of the two surface points a and b. Likewise, $s_a(s_b)$, $e_a(e_b)$, and $c_a(c_b)$ respectively denote the slice value, relative position value of the surface point within the slice, and contour curvature value (given by (5.3)) of the surface point $a(b)$.

5.5.3 Score Matrix Elements

The elements of the score matrix $SC(A, B)$ are computed as a linear combination of the inverse Hausdorff distance and the surface matching score:

$$SC(A, B) = \lambda_1 H^{-1}(A, B) + \lambda_2 FS(A, B), \tag{5.7}$$

where the coefficients of the linear combination are determined using the following constraints:

$$\begin{aligned}
&\lambda_1 + \lambda_2 = 1, \\
&\frac{\lambda_1}{\sigma(H^{-1}(A, B))} = \frac{\lambda_2}{\sigma(FS(A, B))}.
\end{aligned} \tag{5.8}$$

In (5.8), $\sigma(H^{-1}(A, B))$ and $\sigma(FS(A, B))$ respectively denote the standard deviation of the terms $H^{-1}(A, B)$ and $FS(A, B)$ for all possible fracture surface pairs A and B. Let us denote the number of fracture surfaces by n_s and enumerate the fracture surfaces as $1, 2, \ldots, n_s$. The key properties of the score matrix for a multiple-fracture scenario under the assumed configuration, i.e., two fracture surfaces per nonterminal fragment and one fracture surface per terminal fragment, are as follows:

1. The score matrix is *real symmetric*.
2. For two fracture surfaces k and $(k + 1)$ belonging to the same nonterminal fragment, $SC[k][k+1] = 0$, i.e., two fracture surfaces from the same fragment cannot match each other.
3. The diagonal elements of the score matrix are zero, i.e., $SC[k][k] = 0$, i.e., no score is assigned for matching a fracture surface k to itself.
4. In the presence of one or more nonterminal fragments, i.e., two or more nonterminal fracture surfaces, the two fracture surfaces belonging to the two terminal fragments cannot match, i.e., $SC[1][n_s] = 0$.

5.6 Identification of Opposable Fracture Surfaces

In this section, we first derive an expression showing the exponential behavior of the number of reconstruction options to the current reconstruction problem with respect to the number of bone fragments. Next, using the Maximum Weight Graph Matching (MWGM) algorithm, we show how we can identify the juxtaposable fracture surface pairs in polynomial time.

5.6.1 Combinatorial Nature of the Reconstruction Problem

Theorem 5.1 *Given that a nonterminal fragment has two fracture surfaces and a terminal fragment has one fracture surface, the number of possible reconstruction options r_n, where n is the total number of fragments, is $r_n = (n - 2)!2^{(n-2)}$.*

Proof With n total fragments, we have $(n - 2)$ nonterminal fragments and two terminal fragments. The $(n - 2)$ nonterminal fragments can be encountered in any of $(n - 2)!$ possible orderings. Furthermore, each nonterminal fragment can be oriented so that either of the fracture surfaces is the first surface in the sequence. This accounts for the factor $2^{(n-2)}$ in counting the possibilities. □

The presence of a factorial and an exponential term in the above expression for r_n clearly demonstrates the combinatorial nature of the reconstruction problem in terms of the number of reconstruction options. Thus, an exhaustive search for the identification of the opposable fracture surfaces quickly becomes impractical. Note that even for such a reasonably small number of fragments as 6, the number of reconstruction options is 384. It is important to mention that the analysis under the assumption of two fracture surfaces *per* nonterminal fragment and one fracture surface *per* terminal fragment is easily generalized when the above assumptions are relaxed.

5.6.2 Maximum Weight Graph Matching for Restricting the Reconstruction Options

As mentioned in the literature review, various algorithmic and computational geometry-based approaches have been undertaken to restrict the number of reconstruction options for the jigsaw puzzle problem. We use the *Maximum Weight Graph Matching* (MWGM) algorithm to achieve this goal by generating k solution sets, where $k \geq 2$, and the solution sets are indexed by $j, j = 1, \ldots, k$. Recall Theorem 2.3 on the time complexity of the MWGM algorithm. We now state and justify the following claim regarding the modeling of the current reconstruction problem as an MWGM problem.

Claim 5.1 *The Maximum Weight Graph Matching (MWGM) algorithm for a weighted graph correctly identifies, in polynomial time, a number of solution sets, where each individual solution set, given by a collection of unordered opposable fracture surface pairs, is guaranteed to include all the fracture surfaces.*

Justification The fracture surfaces are modeled as the vertices of a weighted graph $G = (V, E)$. The anatomical constraints preclude placement of edges between certain pairs of vertices. We can assign these edges a zero edge weight. The precomputed real symmetric score matrix elements SC_{AB} (from (5.7)), where A and B denote any two fracture surfaces, are assigned positive edge weights w_{AB}. The goal is to identify the sets of opposable fracture surfaces such that the sum of the matching scores is maximized. Thus, the current reconstruction problem maps to the following well-known Maximum Weight Graph Matching (MWGM) problem in graph theory, i.e., given a weighted undirected graph $G = (V, E)$ with edge weights $w_{AB} \geq 0$, obtain a pairing of the vertices such that the sum of the edge weights $\sum w_{AB}$ is maximized. The number of vertices of our graph is even, and hence a complete or perfect matching is guaranteed, i.e., all the opposable fracture surfaces will be included in the fracture surface pairings associated with a solution set. Furthermore, since the score matrix is symmetrical and the graph is undirected, the ordering within an individual pair of surfaces does not matter. At the beginning, we run the MWGM algorithm with the precomputed score matrix. After the (first) solution set is obtained, we modify the score matrix by assigning zero weights to each matrix element whose indices appear in the above solution set. The MWGM algorithm now runs with the modified score matrix and generates a new solution set, which is orthogonal to the previous solution set, and so on. It is imperative that each successive mutually orthogonal (i.e., disjoint) solution set generated by the MWGM algorithm, in this manner, results in a decrease in the value of $\sum w_{AB}$ compared to the previous solution. Let the sum of the edge weights in two successive solutions j and $(j+1)$ be denoted by $(\sum w^j_{AB})$ and $(\sum w^{j+1}_{AB})$, respectively. We continue to generate k solution sets from the MWGM algorithm unless the following constraint is violated:

$$\left(\sum w^j_{AB} - \sum w^{j+1}_{AB}\right) < p \sum w^j_{AB}, \tag{5.9}$$

where p is an appropriately chosen positive constant (0.1 for the present problem). From Theorem 2.3, the MWGM algorithm for a weighted graph G with n vertices (i.e., $n = |V|$), has $O(n^4)$ run-time complexity. If we generate k orthogonal solution sets satisfying (5.9), where k is usually much less than n, then the run-time complexity of our proposed solution is $O(kn^4)$, which is polynomial in n. □

5.7 Pairwise Registration of the Fracture Surfaces

The solution obtained from the MWGM algorithm is a set of pairs of fracture surfaces. Thus, the multiple-fracture registration problem can be viewed as a series of single fracture registration problems. In the previous chapter, we have already discussed several algorithms that can perform single fracture registration. Here, we use the ICP algorithm for pairwise registration of the fracture surfaces. As discussed earlier, the surface point correspondences for any given pair of fracture surfaces are determined using the MCMW bipartite graph matching algorithm [33]. The MCMW bipartite graph matching algorithm obviates the need for any prior alignment of the two fracture surface data sets when computing the *closest set* in the ICP algorithm. We request the reader to revisit Sect. 4.5.1. The entire contents of Sect. 4.5.1, including Theorem 2.2 and Claim 4.1, hold for the pairwise registration of the fracture surfaces in a multiple-fracture scenario.

5.8 Shape Monitoring of the Reconstructed Mandible

Note that we have thus far used (a) a score matrix that is formulated in a manner that is favorable to an optimal solution and (b) a nongreedy MWGM algorithm to solve the problem of multiple-fracture reconstruction. In this section, we exploit the knowledge of the global shape of a human mandible to monitor and verify the reconstruction process at each step. The published literature on automated jigsaw puzzle assembly includes such a verification or validation procedure. For example, Burdea and Wolfson [111] discuss robotic verification of a jigsaw puzzle assembly following the employment of machine vision and combinatorial optimization algorithms. Our overall strategy for solving the multiple-fracture reconstruction problem bears some resemblance to their approach.

Using the MWGM algorithm in the manner described in Sect. 5.6.2, we generate multiple solution sets where each solution set is a collection of fracture surface pairs. The overall verification approach is to start with the best solution set and perform shape checking after every additional fracture surface pair has been registered. At any stage in the reconstruction procedure, if the shape matching constraints are violated, we abandon the current solution set and restart the registration procedure with the next best solution set within the set of orthogonal solutions generated by the MWGM algorithm. Since the desired outcome of the reconstruction is known a priori, we can actually use the desired outcome, or a close approximation thereof, as a reference. For our purpose, we use an unbroken human jaw as a reference shape. We compare the partially reconstructed jaw at every stage of the reconstruction procedure with the unbroken reference jaw.

There are several shape matching algorithms described in the computer vision literature [112, 113]. We employ two constraints based on the Tanimoto coefficient [114] in the context of volumetric shape matching. The Tanimoto coefficient $TC_{f,g}$ between two volumetric shapes f and g is defined as follows [114]:

$$TC_{f,g} = O_{f,g}/(I_f + I_g - O_{f,g}), \tag{5.10}$$

where

$$I_f = \iiint f^2(\hat{x}, \hat{y}, \hat{z})\, dx\, dy\, dz, \tag{5.11}$$

$$I_g = \iiint g^2(\tilde{x}, \tilde{y}, \tilde{z})\, dx\, dy\, dz, \tag{5.12}$$

$$O_{f,g} = 2\iiint f(\hat{x}, \hat{y}, \hat{z}) g(\tilde{x}, \tilde{y}, \tilde{z})\, dx\, dy\, dz. \tag{5.13}$$

Here $(\hat{x}, \hat{y}, \hat{z}) = (x - x_{RC}, y - y_{RC}, z - z_{RC})$ and $(\tilde{x}, \tilde{y}, \tilde{z}) = (x - x_{SC}, y - y_{SC}, z - z_{SC})$ represent respectively the points of the reference mandible R and the reconstructed mandible S with respect to their individual centroids denoted by (x_{RC}, y_{RC}, z_{RC}) and (x_{SC}, y_{SC}, z_{SC}). Also,

$$f(\hat{x}, \hat{y}, \hat{z}) = \begin{cases} 1 & \text{if } (\hat{x}, \hat{y}, \hat{z}) \in R, \\ 0 & \text{otherwise}, \end{cases} \tag{5.14}$$

$$g(\tilde{x}, \tilde{y}, \tilde{z}) = \begin{cases} 1 & \text{if } (\tilde{x}, \tilde{y}, \tilde{z}) \in S, \\ 0 & \text{otherwise}. \end{cases} \tag{5.15}$$

Now, we state and justify the following claim about the constraints based on volumetric matching using (5.10)–(5.15).

Claim 5.2 *The following two shape constraints based on volumetric matching are sufficient to determine the correctness of the reconstruction procedure at any stage*:

(a) $TC_{f,g}$ *is monotonically nondecreasing in successive stages of the multiple-fracture reconstruction procedure, and*
(b) $2I_g - O_{f,g} \leq 2qI_g$, *where* q *is a small positive number* (*chosen as* 0.01 *for the present problem*).

Justification At each stage of the reconstruction procedure, an additional bone fragment is added to the partially reconstructed mandible thus far. In the ideal case (where S is contained in R), adding a bone fragment to S increases the value of the numerator in the defining equation (5.10) while simultaneously decreasing the value of the denominator. Thus, if $TC_{f,g}$ decreases when a bone fragment is added to S, then it is compelling evidence that the solution set we are working with is wrong and should be abandoned. This provides the justification for constraint (a) described above. Note that the reference mandible remains the same throughout the reconstruction procedure, whereas the reconstructed mandible increases in volume in each successive stage of the multiple-fracture reconstruction procedure. Furthermore, note that both, the reference mandible and the reconstructed mandible under consideration, are binary objects. It is quite evident from (5.10)–(5.15) that at any stage, the extent of the volumetric overlap O_{fg} should be exactly twice the reconstructed volume I_g, in the ideal case (where S is contained in R). Thus, for a nonideal solution set to be considered satisfactory, we expect that the inequality $1 - O_{fg}/2I_g < q$ should hold for a small value of q (chosen as 0.01 for the present problem). Multiplying both sides of the inequality by $2I_g$, we get the desired constraint (b) described above. □

5.9 Experimental Results

A salient feature of the virtual multiple-fracture reconstruction problem is its combinatorial pattern matching aspect. The primary emphasis of the work described in this chapter is to show how the MWGM algorithm can be employed to solve this combinatorial pattern matching problem efficiently. It is relevant to mention that segmentation of broken fragments in more complex multiple-fracture situations represents an important though independent problem that is beyond the purview of the work presented in this chapter. Each of the papers [87, 88], and [91] shows experimental results on one or two test cases. For the purpose of experimentation, we have chosen a typical multiple-fracture CT image sequence consisting of six broken bone fragments and altogether ten fracture surfaces, as shown in Fig. 5.2. After the initial image processing tasks of thresholding, connected component labeling, and area-based filtering are performed, the six broken bone fragments are separated (Figs. 5.3 and 5.4). The two fracture surfaces belonging to the terminal fragments are numbered 1 and 10, and the remaining eight fracture surfaces belonging to the nonterminal fragments are numbered from 2 to 9 as shown in Fig. 5.5.

Table 5.1 shows the extreme values amongst the elements of the score matrix *SC*. Recall that *SC* stores the surface matching scores using (5.7) and (5.8) amongst

Table 5.1 Extreme Score Parameter Values

SC Extremes	Value	Fracture Surface Pair
Min. Overall Score	1	$(4, 9)$
Max. Overall Score	1362	$(1, 4)$

Table 5.2 Results from the MWGM algorithm

Solution Set	Score of the solution set
$\{(1,4),(2,5),(3,6),(7,8),(9,10)\}$	4987
$\{(1,3),(2,9),(4,6),(5,7),(8,10)\}$	3123

Table 5.3 Result of shape monitoring at various stages of the multiple-fracture reconstruction procedure

Various Stages of Reconstruction	TC_{fg}	$A = \frac{(2I_g - O_{f,g})}{2I_g}$
$(1,4)$ registered	1.08	0
$(1,4),(2,5)$ registered	1.47	0
$(1,4),(2,5),(3,6)$ registered	1.57	0
$(1,4),(2,5),(3,6),(7,8)$ registered	1.69	0
$(1,4),(2,5),(3,6),(7,8),(9,10)$ registered	21.71	0.0003

all possible fracture surface pairs. The higher the value, the better is the compatibility between the corresponding surfaces for the purpose of further registration. Thus, fracture surfaces 1 and 4 are excellent candidates for registration, whereas it is highly unlikely that fracture surfaces 4 and 9 would be matched together.

Table 5.2 shows the solution set obtained from the MWGM algorithm along with the sum of the edge weights for each solution. Note that each solution is a collection of matching surface pairs. We choose $p = 0.1$ in (5.9), which, in this case, results in the termination of the MWGM algorithm after obtaining two orthogonal solution sets. As the score of the first solution is much higher than that of the second, we cannot expect more competing solutions. The solution pattern clearly demonstrates the effectiveness of the designed score matrix in being able to yield the optimal solution.

Note that the number of reconstruction possibilities for this test case is theoretically derived to be 384 (Sect. 5.6.1). The MWGM algorithm demonstrates that an effective reconstruction can be obtained by exploring just two solutions. On a 1.73-GHz Pentium machine, generation of the solution sets (representing various opposable fracture surface pairs as shown in Table 5.2) takes well less than 1 minute. Figure 5.6 depicts the various stages of mandibular reconstruction corresponding to the best solution of the MWGM algorithm (obtained from row 1 of Table 5.2) using the ICP algorithm described in Sect. 4.5.1. The first row shows three successive images in the original CT sequence with six broken bone fragments or components (denoted by bright intensity values), obtained after preprocessing the original CT image sequence. Each of the later five rows shows the same three images with a new pair of fracture surfaces registered at each stage.

Table 5.3 describes the results at the end of each step of the procedure for monitoring the shape of the partially reconstructed mandible at various stages of multiple-fracture reconstruction. At each stage, both shape constraints (defined in Claim 5.2 in Sect. 5.8) are imposed with a choice of $q = 0.01$ (constraint (b) in Claim 5.2).

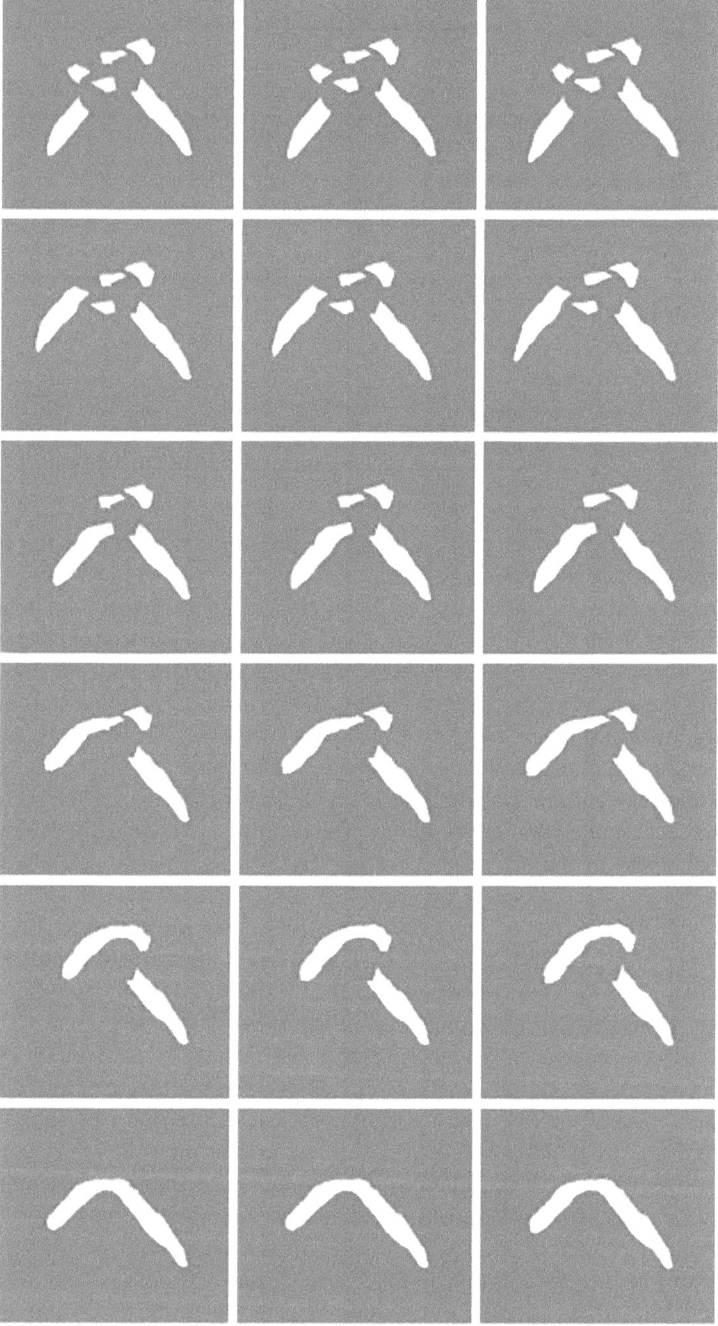

Fig. 5.6 Different stages of multiple-fracture reconstruction as seen in three successive CT image slices

Thus, we proceed with the best solution of the MWGM algorithm to complete the registration of all five fracture surface pairs. Rows 2–4 of Table 5.3 show that the value of TC_{fg} increases by a relatively small amount when a fragment, which is relatively small in volume, is getting added to the partially reconstructed mandible. In the last step of the reconstruction, when a terminal fragment with much larger volume is added to the partially reconstructed mandible via registration of the fracture surfaces 9 and 10, the value of TC_{fg} increases significantly. This is also evident from Fig. 5.6.

5.10 Conclusion and Future Work

We have addressed an important surgical problem of virtual multiple-fracture craniofacial reconstruction within the broader area of biomedical pattern analysis. The problem is appealing from both an application standpoint and a theoretical perspective. From an application standpoint, the fast and accurate reconstruction of fractured human mandible from several broken fragments poses a severe challenge to a practicing surgeon. On the other hand, from a theoretical perspective the problem clearly resembles that of 3D jigsaw puzzle assembly, which, in turn, entails significant combinatorial pattern matching. We have employed computer vision and graph matching algorithms to solve this extremely challenging problem.

In our approach, a score matrix is first constructed using a linear combination of the inverse Hausdorff distance and a function based on contour curvature. Next, an MWGM algorithm is used to identify the opposable fracture surface pairs. The individual fracture surface pairs are registered using an MCMW bipartite graph matching algorithm. Finally, the overall reconstruction process is continuously monitored using shape constraints based on computation of the Tanimoto coefficient. The proposed solution has the potential to reduce considerably the operative time, operative cost, and patient trauma during actual craniofacial surgery, and the risk of postoperative complications.

An obvious direction for future research is to extend the proposed solution for virtual multiple-fracture craniofacial reconstruction to other areas of reconstructive surgery involving multiple fractures such as orthopedic surgery. Issues related to the segmentation of bone fragments in CT images exhibiting complex multiple fractures also need be addressed. We also need to investigate computer vision-guided identification of fracture surfaces and subsequent extraction of fracture surface data to make the proposed virtual reconstruction scheme fully automated.

Part III
Computer-Aided Fracture Detection

Chapter 6
Fracture Detection Using Bayesian Inference

6.1 Motivation

Introducing automation in the various aspects of reconstructive craniofacial surgery is a highly demanding and technically challenging task. The automatic detection of fracture surfaces, which subsequently serve as input data to the surface matching and virtual reconstruction algorithms, is a critical and integral aspect of this endeavor [54, 107]. The generation of fracture surface data thus far has entailed significant user involvement. The surgeon has had to explicitly identify and manually extract the stable fracture points in the CT image sequence of the fractured craniofacial skeleton. This has proved to be a performance bottleneck in attaining the ultimate goal of *in silico* surgery with minimal user intervention. Semi-automatic detection reduces considerably the time and cost of the operation. More importantly, reduced time in the operating room results in reduced operative trauma to the patient and reduced risk for potential postoperative complications.

In this chapter, we present techniques from computer vision and Bayesian statistics to detect stable fracture points in Computed Tomography (CT) image sequences of a human mandible upon having experienced craniofacial trauma. The fracture patterns under consideration are typically characterized by bone fragments that are well displaced and are termed as well-displaced or major fractures. A two-phase semi-automatic scheme for reliable detection and accurate localization of stable fracture points is proposed. In the first phase, an initial pool of fracture points is obtained by detecting points of high curvature on the contours of the broken mandibular fragments. Several of the false positives are filtered out using length and orientation constraints on a cycle graph-based representation of the detected fracture points. In the second phase, only anatomically correct fracture points are retained by enforcing spatial consistency constraints amongst the existing fracture points using a Kalman filter formulated within a Bayesian inference framework.

The approach described in this chapter is shown to reduce considerably the user intervention required in the detection of stable fracture points. The only user inputs required are the length and orientation bounds for a potential fracture in a given dataset. In addition to its obvious practical benefit in terms of enabling an important

A.S. Chowdhury, S.M. Bhandarkar, *Computer Vision-Guided Virtual Craniofacial Surgery*, Advances in Computer Vision and Pattern Recognition,
DOI 10.1007/978-0-85729-296-4_6,

biomedical imaging application, i.e., virtual craniofacial surgery, the work presented in this chapter has some points of theoretical novelty as well. The Kalman filter, used to verify the spatial consistency of the observed fracture points, is formulated within a Bayesian inference framework. Note that the Kalman filter, in its canonical form, essentially predicts the value of a future state (position of a fracture point in the context of the present work) given the present state and the past states. We show here how a limited reliable zone of prediction can be formulated using *Credible Sets* within a Bayesian formulation. The main challenges behind this work are summarized below:

(a) A fracture point is equivalent to a corner. But a simple corner detection algorithm detects many spurious corners or anatomically incorrect fracture points. This is due to the presence of soft tissue, cavities, and rugged contours of the broken mandibular fragments.
(b) Presence of noise in the CT scans of the mandibles also increases the level of difficulty of the problem.
(c) Specifications of mere point estimates of the fracture points in various slices are not always enough to check the consistency, especially given the lower resolution along the axial direction (Z-axis) and the presence of noise.

6.2 Chapter Organization

The overall organization of this chapter is as follows: Sect. 6.3 presents the related work and highlights our contribution. Section 6.4 describes the initial image processing tasks that are performed prior to fracture surface detection. The details of the image processing tasks are omitted to avoid repetition, and the reader is requested to revisit Sect. 4.4 for details. Section 6.5 illustrates the detection of potential fracture points in individual 2D CT image slices. Section 6.5 contains two subsections, where Sect. 6.5.1 discusses the determination of the initial pool of fracture points. Section 6.5.2 discusses the methods used to filter out incorrect fracture points and retain the potentially valid ones. Section 6.6 describes the detection of anatomically stable fracture points across the 2D CT image slices that constitute a given CT image sequence. Like the previous section, Sect. 6.6 also comprises of two subsections. Sect. 6.6.1 discusses the formulation of a Kalman filter within a Bayesian inference framework, whereas Sect. 6.6.2 establishes the concept of spatial consistency of the detected fracture points. In Sect. 6.7, we present the experimental results. The chapter is concluded in Sect. 6.8 with an outline for future research directions.

6.3 Related Work and Our Contribution

In this section, we first discuss various existing techniques for automatic fracture detection in CT and X-ray images and then highlight the novel aspects of our proposed scheme. Existing published literature on fracture detection in CT and X-ray images describes the use of various approaches such as a *divide-and-conquer* approach combined with the exploitation of anatomical knowledge for the detection of hip fractures by Ozanian and Philips [115]; a texture analysis-based approach for the detection of hip fractures by Yap et al. [116]; an approach that combines adaptive interface agents with neural networks to detect fractures in long bones by Syiam et al. [117]; a probabilistic approach based on a combination of various statistical classifiers for the detection of fractures in femur bones by Lum et al. [118]; active contour modeling coupled with shape constraints for the detection of fractures in the arm by Jia and Jiang [119]; femur fracture detection via a divide-and-conquer approach in kernel-space using a Support Vector Machine (SVM) by He et al. [120], and the use of the Hough transform and gradient analysis for the detection of mid-shaft long bone fractures by Donnelley et al. [121].

Although mandibular fractures are encountered frequently, there is a relative dearth of research work in computer-aided detection of such fractures. Now, we explain the various choices and tradeoffs involved in the formulation and design of our scheme for automated mandibular fracture detection and localization in a CT image sequence. We also state and justify the salient features and advantages of our scheme in the context of aformentioned works. We exploit anatomical knowledge in a manner similar to [115]. However, the *divide-and-conquer approach*, discussed therein [115], is not particularly useful for our problem. From our CT image data we have made a careful observation that the pixel intensity values, shape constraints, and anatomical knowledge are important factors to be considered, but not the image texture. Thus, the approach outlined in [116] is not applicable. We do not use a neural network-based approach, as outlined in [117] or an SVM-based approach, like [120], because, thus far, there is no learning component involved in this problem. In addition, we want to ensure that the execution time of the proposed method is low, which is often seen to be a problem in a neural network-based approach. As we are interested in detecting fracture points, a Hough transform-based solution, as described in [121], is not very relevant. Isolation of anatomically correct fracture points from the incorrect ones can be formulated as a classification problem. However, we take a simple yet novel threshold-based approach (described in more detail in Sect. 6.5) instead of a relatively complex approach based on the combination of probabilistic classifiers [118]. Note that we incorporate the notion of probabilistic detection in a different manner by statistically modeling the Kalman filter. Last, but not the least, we employ shape constraints in a manner similar to [119]. But, instead of using an active contour model, we model and check the spatial consistency of a fracture point.

A flowchart of the proposed multi-fracture reconstruction scheme is shown in Fig. 6.1. As mentioned earlier, the proposed approach works well for the class of well-displaced fractures. Initial image processing tasks, such as entropy thresholding and connected component labeling, are performed on 2D slices. A novel two-phase semi-automatic scheme for detection of stable fracture points is carried out next. In the first phase, an initial pool of fracture points is obtained by detecting points of high curvature on the contours of the broken mandibular bone fragments. Many false positives are filtered out using length and ori-

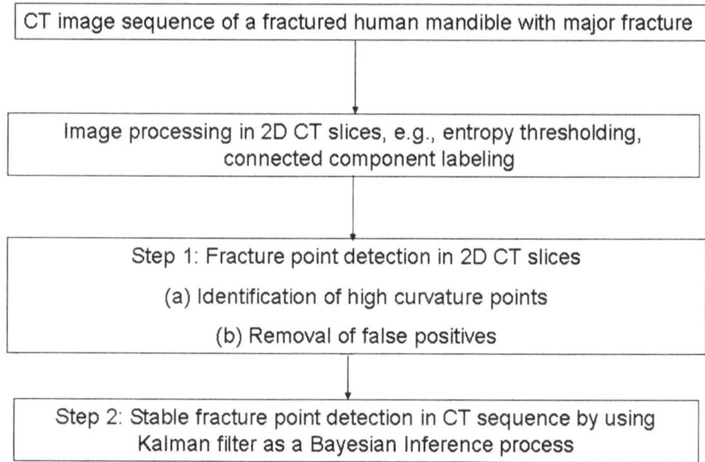

Fig. 6.1 Flowchart for major fracture detection

entation constraints on a cycle graph-based representation of the detected fracture points. In the second phase, only anatomically correct fracture points are retained by imposing spatial consistency constraints amongst the existing fracture points and propagating these constraints across the 2D CT image slices using the standard Kalman filter [122] formulated within a Bayesian inference framework [123]. We show in this paper how a limited reliable zone of prediction can be formulated using *Credible Sets* within a Bayesian formulation. A new figure-of-merit term, based on 95% and 99% Bayesian prediction intervals, is introduced as a measure of anatomical correctness for the detected fracture points. From an application perspective, the work presented in this chapter constitutes a crucial and integral part of a virtual craniofacial reconstruction scheme. The approach undertaken in this work reduces considerably the user intervention needed in the detection of anatomically correct fracture points in the fractured mandible. Some part of the work described in this chapter has appeared in [124].

6.4 Image Processing

The image processing consists of thresholding and connected component labeling. In the case of phantom data, a simple thresholding scheme is sufficient. For real patient data, on the other hand, entropy-based thresholding is employed to obtain better results. Standard image processing operations such as connected component labeling followed by area-based (size) filtering are performed on the thresholded images. In the interest of avoiding needless repetition, the details are omitted here; the reader can revisit Sect. 4.4 for these details. However, Figs. 6.2 and 6.3 are repeated from Sect. 4.4 for the sake of completeness. A typical result of the aforementioned

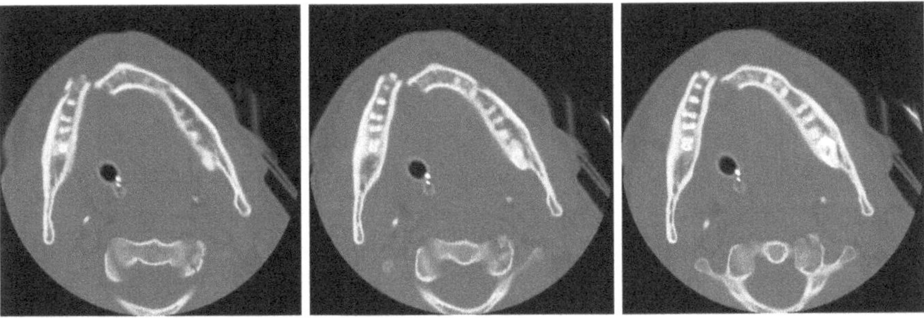

Fig. 6.2 A real patient CT image sequence of a fractured mandible. The images in (**a**), (**b**), and (**c**) are three consecutive slices in the CT sequence

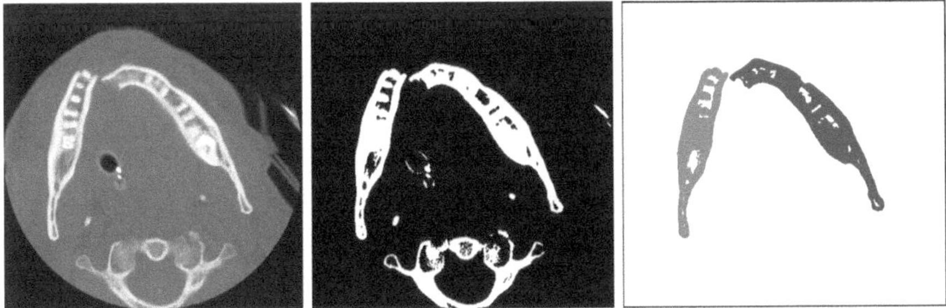

Fig. 6.3 (**a**) A typical 2D CT slice from a real patient CT sequence. (**b**) The CT slice after entropy-based thresholding. (**c**) The CT slice after connected component labeling and size filtering. In (**c**), the two broken mandibular fragments are represented by two different intensity values

image processing operations on a single CT image slice is depicted in Fig. 6.3(c). The processed CT image slices are then used for identification and localization of fracture points.

6.5 Fracture Point Detection in 2D CT Image Slices

In the first phase of the proposed scheme, we detect the fracture points in the individual 2D CT image slices. This is accomplished broadly in two steps. In the first step, an initial pool of potential fracture points is obtained by detecting points of high curvature on the contours of the broken mandibular fragments. In the second step, the potential fracture points on a component (i.e., bone fragment) in a CT image slice are modeled as a cycle graph. A final pool of potential fracture points is selected by coalescing the closely spaced points and filtering out some additional points based on certain predefined geometric constraints.

6.5.1 Initial Pool of Fracture Points

As mentioned earlier, a fracture point is essentially a point of high curvature. Hence, we use a simple corner point detection technique to generate an initial pool of high-curvature points or corners. Throughout the rest of the chapter, the terms *fracture point*, *high-curvature point*, and *corner point* will be used synonymously. We follow the simple approach for corner point detection outlined in [125]. This method of corner point detection is based on estimation of the tangent orientation using edge points that are not adjacent in the edge list *EL*. Let $|EL|$ be the total number of edge pixels of a 2D component, $EL[i]$ be the ith pixel in the edge list *EL*, k be the number of forward and backward edge pixels used to determine whether the pixel i is a potential corner, ϕ_{ij} be the angle between any two edge pixels i and j, and θ be the threshold angle for corner determination. Note that the value of k determines the scale at which the local curvature at an edge point is computed. True corner points can be expected to exhibit sufficiently high curvature values over a substantial range of k (i.e., scale) values. The following algorithm is used to detect corner points [125]:

```
for i ∈ [1, |EL|]
    for m ∈ [1, k]
        Find φ_{i+m,i−m} ;
        if (|φ_{i+m,i−m}| > θ)
            continue ;
        else
            break ;
        end if ;
    end for ;
    if ∀m, (|φ_{i+m,i−m}| > θ)
        mark i as a fracture point ;
    end if ;
end for ;
```

Let c be the number of components. Then, the time complexity of the above algorithm can be shown to be $O(ck|EL|)$.

6.5.2 Final Pool of Fracture Points

By treating each corner as a vertex and assuming an edge between each successive pair of corners, a weighted cycle graph $G(V, E)$ is generated for each component in each 2D CT image slice. The weight of an edge connecting a pair of vertices is the Euclidean distance between the corresponding corner points. Closely spaced vertices are coalesced and a corresponding subgraph $G_1(V_1, E_1)$ is constructed. Next, based on a prior knowledge of the range of length and orientation values of an edge that could connect two potential fracture points; a smaller subgraph $G_2(V_2, E_2)$ is constructed. Note that the lower and upper bounds on the length and orientation values of a fracture edge are different for different CT image sequences. After the above filtering operations are performed, we are left with a smaller and more likely pool of fracture points. The combined time complexity of the above two filtering operations is $O(|E|) + O(|E_1|)$.

6.6 Stable Fracture Points in a CT Image Sequence

In the second phase of our scheme, we establish the spatial consistency of the detected corner points across the CT image slices that constitute a given CT image sequence. Successive 2D CT image slices of a given 3D object can be modeled as observations at different time instants. Consequently, we can track the detected fracture points along successive 2D CT image slices. We develop a mathematical criterion of spatial consistency, which is analogous to the temporal consistency criterion used in most tracking algorithms for dynamic or time-elapsed images.

6.6.1 The Kalman Filter as a Bayesian Inference Process

We first introduce the standard Kalman filter following [122] and then explain how it can be treated as a Bayesian inference problem using [123] and [126]. The Kalman filter is an efficient recursive filter that estimates the state of a linear dynamic system from a series of noisy measurements. The Kalman filter has found wide acceptance in control theory, computer vision, image processing, and signal processing. A common application of the Kalman filter in computer vision and image processing is the tracking of an object or target in a temporal sequence of images (i.e., a video stream). The individual images in the video stream typically contain a sequence of noisy observations about the position of a target. The Kalman filter is used to provide accurate and continuously updated information about the position and the velocity of the target from these noisy observations. In a Kalman filter, the state and measurement vectors for a target at a time t are given by the following linear stochastic difference equations [122]:

$$X_t = AX_{t-1} + w_t, \tag{6.1}$$

$$Z_t = HX_t + v_t. \tag{6.2}$$

Here $X_t \in \Re^2$ denotes the actual state or parameter vector, and $Z_t \in \Re^2$ denotes the measurement or observation vector. The matrix A in (6.1) relates the state vector at the previous time step $(t-1)$ to the state vector at the current time step t. Similarly, the matrix H in (6.2) relates the state vector to the measurement vector. In the context of the present problem, both A and H are considered to be 2×2 identity matrices. We further assume both the process noise w_t and the measurement noise v_t to be normally distributed with zero mean and constant variance Q and R, respectively, i.e.,

$$p(w) \sim \mathcal{N}(0, Q), \tag{6.3}$$
$$p(v) \sim \mathcal{N}(0, R). \tag{6.4}$$

Under the assumption that the initial state vector X_0 is normal with mean μ_0 and variance Σ_0, let us define:

$$\begin{aligned} \mu_{t-1} &= E\big[X_{t-1} \mid Z^{t-1}\big], \\ \Sigma_{t-1} &= \text{var}\big[X_{t-1} \mid Z^{t-1}\big], \end{aligned} \tag{6.5}$$

where $Z^{t-1} = [Z_1, \ldots, Z_{t-1}]$. It is important to note that the Kalman filter leads to a recursive procedure for inference about the state vector X_t. Thus, given the data (measurement) vector $\hat{Z}_t$, inference about X_t can be derived following the well-known Bayes' theorem [123]:

Prob.(State of Nature|Data)

$\propto$ Prob(Data|State of Nature) $\times$ Prob.(State of Nature),

which can be mathematically written as

$$P\big(X_t \mid Z^t\big) \propto P\big(Z^t \mid X_t, Z^{t-1}\big) \times P\big(X_t \mid Z^{t-1}\big). \tag{6.6}$$

In the above equation, the term on the left side represents the *posterior* distribution of X at time t, while the first and second terms on the right side represent the *likelihood* distribution and *prior* distribution for X, respectively. The prior distribution can be written as [126]

$$\big(X_t \mid Z^{t-1}\big) \sim \mathcal{N}(\mu_{t-1}, \Sigma_{t-1} + Q). \tag{6.7}$$

The likelihood distribution is given by [126]

$$\big(Z_t \mid X_t, Z^{t-1}\big) \sim \mathcal{N}(\mu_{t-1}, \Sigma_{t-1} + Q + R). \tag{6.8}$$

Based on the prior distribution and the likelihood distribution given above, the posterior distribution can be expressed as [126]

$$\big(X_t \mid Z^t\big) \sim \mathcal{N}\big(\mu_{t-1} + KF_t(Z_t - \mu_{t-1}), KF_t R\big). \tag{6.9}$$

Here, KF_t is called the Kalman filter gain and is given by

$$KF_t = (\Sigma_{t-1} + Q)(\Sigma_{t-1} + Q + R)^{-1}. \tag{6.10}$$

Note that the posterior mean $(\mu_{t-1} + KF_t(Z_t - \mu_{t-1}))$ in (6.9) is equal to the prior mean (μ_{t-1}) from (6.8) plus an update term involving the Kalman filter gain KF_t given by (6.10).

6.6.2 Concept of Spatial Consistency

Statistical confidence measures have been used widely in various image processing and computer vision problems including those in the domain of medical imaging. Examples of the use of statistical confidence measures can be found in the works of Ye et al. for analyzing and visualizing the performance of two-dimensional parametric shape estimators [127], Subramanian et al. for interactive detection and visualization of images of breast lesions from Dynamic Contrast Enhanced Magnetic Resonance Images (DCE-MRI) [128], and Simonson et al. for binary image registration [129], among several others. In this paper, we use statistical confidence regions for detecting anatomically stable fracture points in a given CT image sequence. The spatial consistency criterion is developed by introducing the concept of Bayesian prediction intervals. We prove the following lemmas about the proposed Bayesian prediction intervals:

Lemma 6.1 *The posterior predictive distribution* $(\tilde{Z}_t|Z_t)$ *is given by* $(\tilde{Z}_t|Z_t) \sim \mathcal{N}(\mu_{t-1} + KF_t(Z_t - \mu_{t-1}), (KF_t + I)R)$.

Proof It can be shown, following Gelman et al. [130], that the posterior predictive distribution has the same mean as the posterior distribution, whereas its variance is equal to the sum of the prior predictive variance of the model and the variance of the posterior distribution. Thus, from (6.9) it follows that the posterior predictive mean is given by $\mu_{t-1} + KF_t(Z_t - \mu_{t-1})$, whereas from (6.9) and (6.4) it follows that the posterior predictive variance is given by $(KF_t + I)R$, where I is an identity matrix. □

Lemma 6.2 *For the independent univariate case, a* $100(1-\alpha)\%$ *credible prediction square for the state vector* X_t *is given by*

$$\mu_{i(t-1)} + KF_{it}(Z_{it} - \mu_{i(t-1)}) \pm z_{\frac{\tau}{2}}\sqrt{(KF_{it} + I)R_{ii}},$$
$$i = 1, 2;\ \tau = 1 - \sqrt{1-\alpha}.$$

Proof Note that for a normal random variable Y with mean η and variance σ^2, we can state the following [131]:

$$P\big[(\eta - \sigma z_{\frac{\tau}{2}}) < Y < (\eta + \sigma z_{\frac{\tau}{2}})\big] = 1 - \tau, \tag{6.11}$$

where z_τ is the upper 100th percentile point of a standard normal distribution. From Lemma 6.1 we can state that the ith component (where $i = 1, 2$, corresponding to the x and y directions, respectively) of $(\tilde{Z}_{it}|Z_{it})$ obeys the following normal distribution:

$$(\tilde{Z}_{it}|Z_{it}) \sim \mathcal{N}\big(\mu_{i(t-1)} + KF_{it}(Z_{it} - \mu_{i(t-1)}), (KF_{it} + I)R_{ii}\big).$$

Since in the a posteriori distribution the components of the state vector are normally and independently distributed, we get:

$$P\big[X_{it} \in \big(\mu_{i(t-1)} + KF_{it}(Z_{it} - \mu_{i(t-1)}) - z_{\frac{\tau}{2}}\sqrt{(KF_{it} + I)R_{ii}},$$
$$\mu_{i(t-1)} + KF_{it}(Z_{it} - \mu_{i(t-1)}) + z_{\frac{\tau}{2}}\sqrt{(KF_{it} + I)R_{ii}}\big),\ i = 1, 2 \,\big|\, Z^t\big]$$
$$= \prod_{i=1}^{2} P\big[X_{it} \in \big(\mu_{i(t-1)} + KF_{it}(Z_{it} - \mu_{i(t-1)}) - z_{\frac{\tau}{2}}\sqrt{(KF_{it} + I)R_{ii}},$$

$$\mu_{i(t-1)} + KF_{it}(Z_{it} - \mu_{i(t-1)}) + z_{\frac{\tau}{2}}\sqrt{(KF_{it} + I)R_{ii}}\big) \mid Z^t\big]$$
$$= (1 - \tau)^2$$
$$= (1 - \alpha).$$ □

Let the Bayesian prediction interval at any time point t along the ith direction be CS_{it}. Then, a fracture point is deemed to be spatially consistent at time point $(t + 1)$ if the following condition is satisfied:

$$Z_{i(t+1)} \in CS_{it} \quad \text{for } i = 1, 2. \tag{6.12}$$

Note that a particular time point in the present context corresponds to a specific image slice in a CT image sequence. In a typical CT image sequence, the fractured mandible appears in a subset of the image slices comprising the entire CT image sequence. Since it is assumed that there is no significant bone deformation, the shape of the fracture pattern does not change dramatically from one CT image slice to the next and changes only gradually over the aforementioned subset of CT image slices. Note that there can be many spurious fracture points detected in the initial pool and some of these may persist after the first phase of the filtering process has been performed. This fact motivates us to perform a spatial consistency check of the observed fracture points across the aforementioned subset of CT image slices. Intuitively, the fracture points which conform to the spatial consistency criterion (6.12) over most of the CT slices in the subset under consideration should be deemed anatomically stable fracture points for the CT image sequence. A figure-of-merit term (S) is introduced for this purpose. Let n be the total number of CT image slices in the aforementioned subset of the original CT image sequence, m be the number of slices in which a particular fracture point is observed, and p be the number of slices in which the fracture point is found to be spatially consistent. Then, S is defined as

$$S = 0.5\big(m/n + p/(m - 1)\big). \tag{6.13}$$

The maximum value of S is unity, which occurs when both m/n and $p/(m - 1)$ attain their maximum value, i.e., unity. The fracture points which yield a high value of S are deemed to be the ones which are anatomically stable and correct. We now explain, in detail, our choice for S. Since the consistency check is performed from the second slice onwards, we have $(m - 1)$ instead of m in the denominator of the second term in (6.13). The second term needs a value of p close to $(m - 1)$ in order for a fracture point to be anatomically stable and correct. It is important to include the first term, i.e., m/n, in the expression for the figure-of-merit term S as well. This is because a fracture point may be found to be consistent in most of the slices in which it appears, which results in a high value of $p/(m - 1)$. However, the same point may appear in only a few slices, which results in a low value of m/n and hence a corresponding low value of S. Thus, we essentially need high values for both the terms in (6.13). The maximum value for each of the two terms in (6.13) could be 1.0, whereas their minimum values could be 0. So, even if one term assumes a maximum and the other term assumes a minimum value, the overall value of S would be 0.5. We deem a corner point to be stable if its figure-of-merit value S exceeds a certain threshold S_{th}. Thus S_{th} should be chosen > 0.5 to ensure that a corner point would be deemed stable if and only if it yields a reasonably high value for both the terms constituting the figure-of-merit S (6.13).

6.7 Experimental Results

In this section, we present the results of the proposed two-phase fracture detection scheme on different CT datasets. We choose $k = 10$ as the value of the scale parameter which essentially determines the number of forward and backward pixels that one needs to consider in order to extract points of high curvature along the contours of the broken bone fragments (see Sect. 6.5.1). The number of potential fracture points resulting from the extraction of such high-curvature points in a typical CT image sequence is found to be unacceptably high. This indicates that a standard corner detector has a tendency to generate a lot of false positives. The potential fracture points for the individual components (i.e., bone fragments) in each CT image slice are modeled as a cycle graph followed by the imposition of the length constraint and orientation constraint on its edges. Typical values of the edge-length bounds (in terms of pixels) and the edge-orientation bounds (in degrees) are $[10, 40]$ and $[50°, 90°]$, respectively. The imposition of the edge-length and edge-orientation constraints results in a significant reduction in the number of anatomically incorrect fracture points. Table 6.1 shows that up to 87% of the initially detected fracture points can be eliminated using the edge-length and edge-orientation constraints. Since imposition of the edge-length and edge-orientation constraints entails user input, the proposed scheme is deemed as one that is semi-automated rather than one that is fully automated.

In the second phase of the proposed scheme, we use a Kalman filter, modeled within a Bayesian inference paradigm, to identify spatially consistent fracture points across all the CT image slices constituting a CT image sequence. We check the consistency of the observed corners using the figure-of-merit term S with 95% and 99% credible sets. It is observed that if we choose a very high value of S_{th}, then spurious fracture points are guaranteed to be eliminated, but there is a potential risk of missing some stable corner points. On the other hand, a low value of S_{th} ensures the detection of true fracture points along with some additional spurious ones. We have already shown that we need a value of S_{th} greater than 0.5 for the detection

Table 6.1 Statistics of the detected fracture points after Phase-I

Dataset	No. of Initial Corners	No. of Corners after Phase-I	% Removed
1	642	136	78.8
2	530	135	74.5
3	848	113	86.7
4	1054	142	86.5
5	747	157	79.0

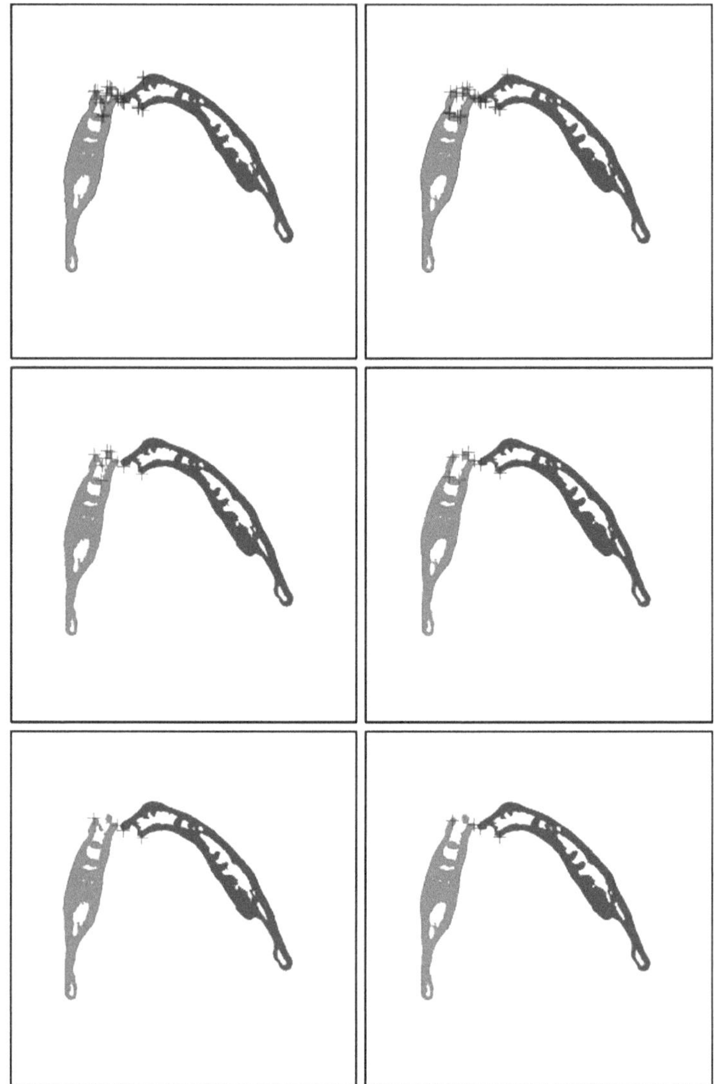

Fig. 6.4 Results of stable fracture point detection for two consecutive CT slices of CT dataset I. The *first row* shows the initially detected fracture points in two successive CT slices; the second row shows the result of filtering using edge-length and edge-orientation constraints (Phase-I); the *third row* shows the consistent corner points obtained using the Bayesian inference procedure (Phase-II). The *centers of the dark crosses* indicate fracture points in each CT slice

of stable and meaningful corner points. Taking into consideration of all the above factors, a value of 0.6 is chosen for S_{th}.

Potential fracture points for two consecutive CT image slices for three different CT datasets are shown in Figs. 6.4, 6.5 and 6.6. We have chosen to show two con-

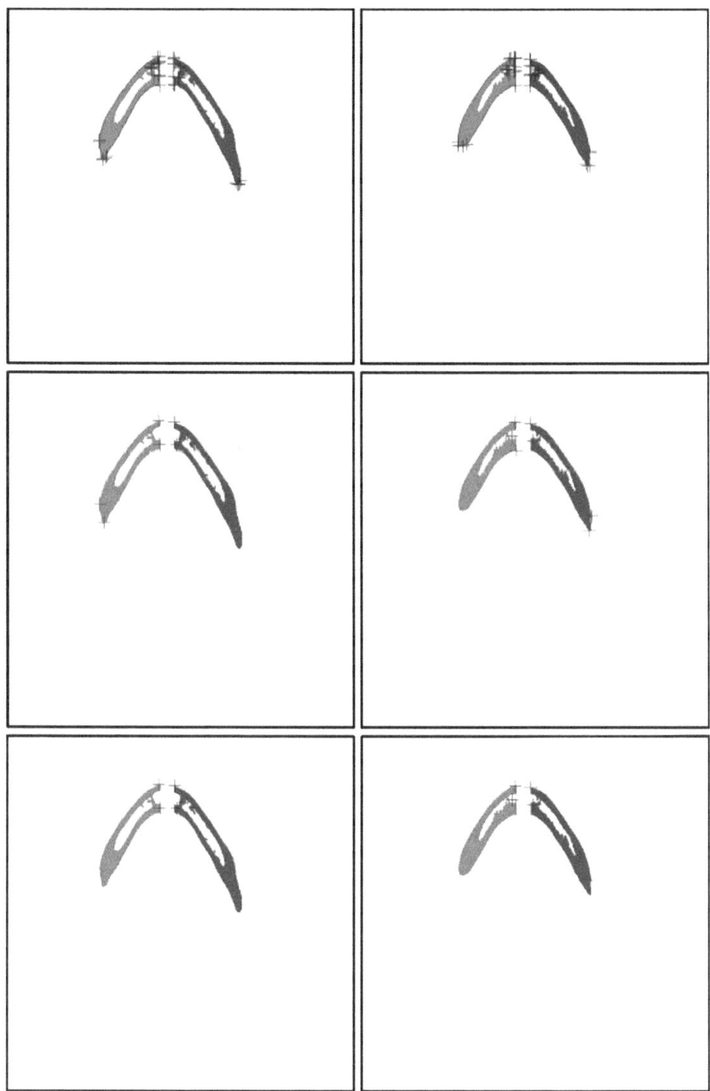

Fig. 6.5 Results of stable fracture detection for two consecutive CT slices of CT dataset II. The *first row* shows the initially detected fracture points in two successive CT slices; the *second row* shows the result of filtering using edge-length and edge-orientation constraints (Phase-I); the *third row* shows the consistent corner points obtained using the Bayesian inference procedure (Phase-II). The *centers of the dark crosses* indicate fracture points in each CT slice

secutive CT image slices solely for the purpose of illustration. A potential fracture point is marked by a dark cross in Figs. 6.4, 6.5 and 6.6. As mentioned in Sect. 6.6.2, the corner points with a value of S greater than S_{th} are deemed to be anatomically stable. In Table 6.2, these corner points are indicated in bold font for all the datasets presented in this section.

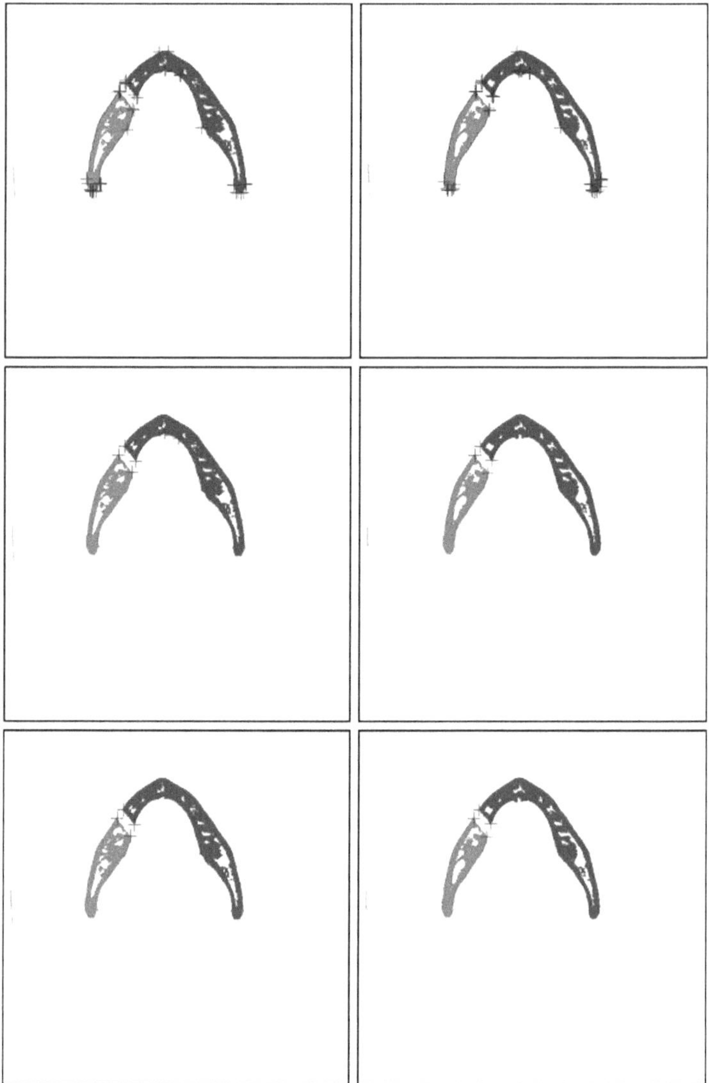

Fig. 6.6 Results of stable fracture detection for two consecutive CT slices of CT dataset III. The *first row* shows the initially detected fracture points in two successive CT slices; the second row shows the result of filtering using edge-length and edge-orientation constraints (Phase-I); the *third row* shows the consistent corner points obtained using the Bayesian inference procedure (Phase-II). The *centers of the dark crosses* indicate fracture points in each CT slice

We observe that between 8 and 13 apparently consistent corner points appear in the 2D CT slices of the input sequences upon completion of Phase-I of the proposed scheme. However, not all of these corner points can be deemed to be anatomically meaningful fracture points. This clearly demonstrates the importance of Phase-II

Table 6.2 Statistics of the detected fracture points after Phase-II. The anatomically stable corner points are denoted using a bold font

Dataset	Corner No.	S (based on 95% CS)	S (based on 99% CS)
Dataset 1	**1**	**0.62**	**0.62**
	2	**0.84**	**0.88**
	3	**0.84**	**0.86**
	4	**0.66**	**0.69**
	5	0.46	0.46
	6	0.04	0.04
	7	0.04	0.54
	8	0.06	0.23
Dataset 2	1	0.39	0.39
	2	0.49	0.49
	3	**0.63**	**0.63**
	4	0.12	0.12
	5	**0.84**	**0.90**
	6	0.09	0.09
	7	**0.88**	**0.90**
	8	**0.90**	**0.93**
	9	0.32	0.46
Dataset 3	**1**	**0.90**	**0.95**
	2	**0.95**	**0.98**
	3	**0.84**	**0.86**
	4	**0.93**	**0.95**
	5	0.49	0.49
	6	0.32	0.32
	7	0.25	0.26
	8	0.56	0.57
Dataset 4	1	0.52	0.55
	2	0.33	0.33
	3	0.45	0.45
	4	**0.85**	**0.90**
	5	0.51	0.51
	6	**0.78**	**0.78**
	7	**0.82**	**0.88**
	8	**0.95**	**0.95**
	9	0.32	0.36

Table 6.2 (*Continued*)

Dataset	Corner No.	*S* (based on 95% CS)	*S* (based on 99% CS)
Dataset 5	1	0.56	0.57
	2	0.55	0.58
	3	0.50	0.50
	4	**1.00**	**1.00**
	5	0.34	0.34
	6	**0.95**	**0.98**
	7	**0.93**	**0.93**
	8	**0.90**	**0.90**
	9	0.30	0.32
	10	0.04	0.04
	11	0.03	0.04
	12	0.04	0.04
	13	0.07	0.09

to further filter out the remaining false positives based on their S values. Recall that S is a figure-of-merit term computed using a Bayesian inference approach (see Sect. 6.6). The value of S remains approximately the same (as expected) when we switch between the computation of 95% and 99% credible sets. In the case of corner 7 in dataset 1, we see a jump in the value of S from 0.04 to 0.54. This sharp change in the value of S is contributed by the second factor in (6.13), more specifically, by a change in the value of p from 0 to 1. Since the higher value of S is still less than S_{th}, the corresponding fracture point is deemed to be unreliable. Table 6.2 shows that most of the anatomically stable corner points possess very high values of S. Furthermore, only 4 corner points in each of the experimental datasets are observed to yield a value of S that is greater than S_{th}. In fact, these 4 corner points are determined to be the only anatomically correct fracture points, upon visual comparison with fracture points that were determined manually. The entire process of fracture detection for a given dataset takes well less than a minute on a 1.73-GHz Intel Pentium-M© processor.

Next, we show a visual comparison between the stable fracture points obtained using the proposed Bayesian inference procedure with those obtained manually for the three experimental datasets depicted in Figs. 6.7, 6.8, and 6.9, respectively. Note that the manual extraction of stable fracture points was performed on the original CT image sequence without any image processing operations, whereas the proposed fracture detection procedure was performed on the broken mandibular fragments after the image processing operations are performed. The above comparison clearly demonstrates the correctness of the proposed method.

Finally, in Table 6.3, we demonstrate quantitatively the accuracy of our proposed method for fracture point extraction by computing the average error and the root-mean-squared (rms) error, both measured in terms of distance (in pixel coordinates) from the manually extracted fracture points. For a specific dataset, we compute the

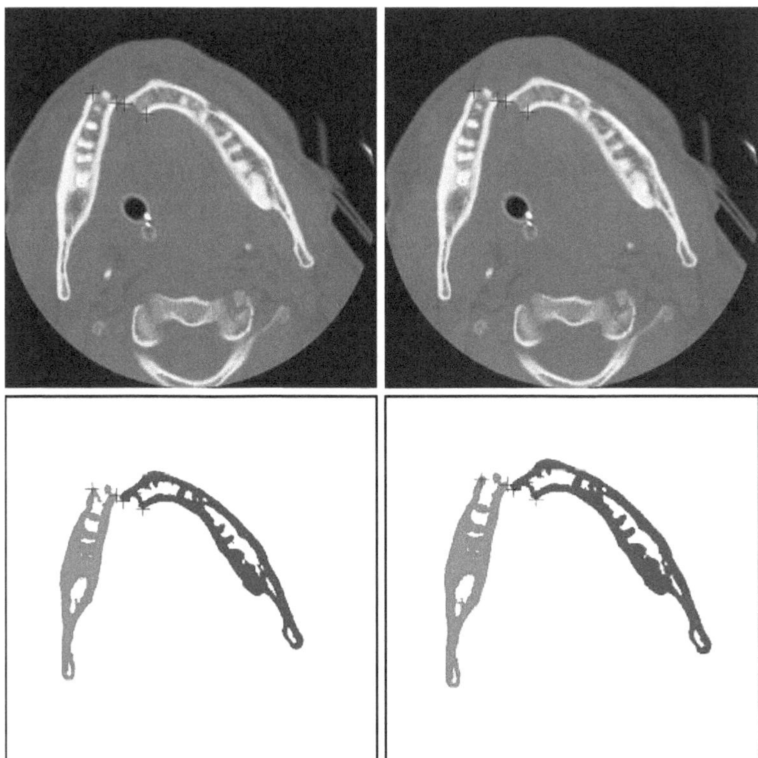

Fig. 6.7 Comparison of stable fracture points detected manually with those detected using the proposed method for two consecutive CT slices of CT dataset-I. The *first row* shows the result of manual fracture point extraction for two consecutive CT slices; the *second row* shows the results of fracture point detection following the Bayesian inference procedure

distance between each stable fracture point, detected by the proposed algorithm, and the corresponding manually extracted fracture point. The average values and the rms values of all the distances (corresponding to all stable fracture points) for the above dataset are computed. Thus, for each dataset, we report an *average error* ± *rms error*. This procedure is repeated for all the experimental datasets. The overall extraction accuracy, computed by taking the average of individual *average errors* and the average of individual *rms errors*, is found to be (2.99 ± 1.69) pixels. As each 2D slice under consideration is 512 pixels wide and 512 pixels high, the surgeons have deemed the estimated error values to be well within the acceptable limit.

6.8 Conclusion and Future Work

In this chapter, a novel, two-phase scheme for semi-automatic detection of mandibular fractures from a CT image sequence is proposed. The class of fracture patterns

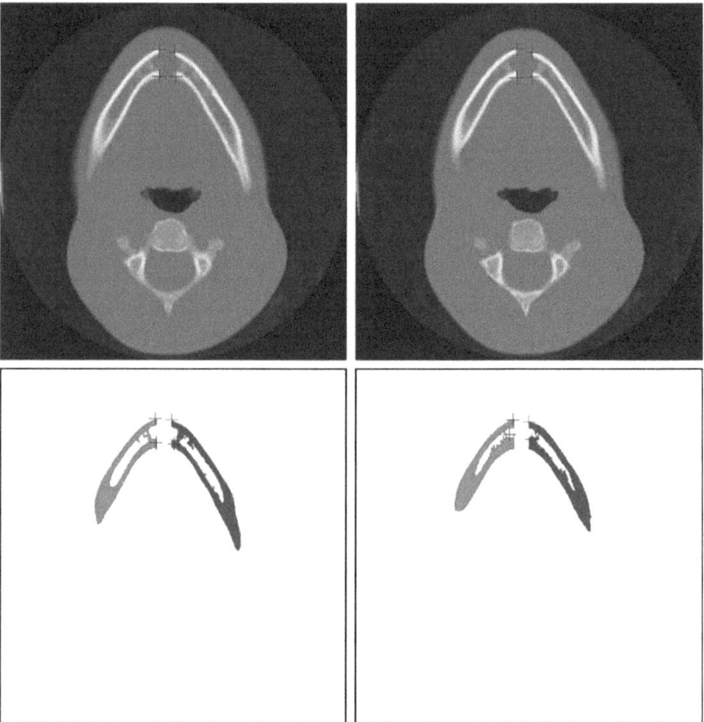

Fig. 6.8 Comparison of stable fracture points detected manually with those detected using the proposed method for two consecutive CT slices of CT dataset-II. The *first row* shows the result of manual fracture point extraction for two consecutive CT slices; the *second row* shows the results of fracture point detection following the Bayesian inference procedure

under consideration consists of well-displaced or clearly broken mandibular fragments. In the first phase of the proposed two-phase approach, an initial pool of high-curvature points is generated. This is followed by a filtering technique that employs length and orientation constraints on the edges of a cycle graph-based representation of the initial pool of fracture points. In the second phase, we use a Kalman filter, viewed from a Bayesian inference perspective, and construct Bayesian prediction intervals for the verification of spatial consistency. A figure-of-merit term is introduced, a high value of which indicates an anatomically stable or correct fracture point. Note that a conventional corner detector can output only a pool of potential corner points in a 2D CT image slice. The false positives in this pool of potential corner points are eliminated efficiently by first using the filtering constraints and then using the Kalman filter to exploit spatial coherence along the axial direction, i.e., across multiple CT image slices. From a biomedical imaging perspective, the contribution of the work described in this chapter lies in enhancing the degree of automation in virtual mandibular surgery. From a theoretical standpoint, the formulation of a figure-of-merit term, accompanied by the specification of a reliable zone for spatial consistency using Bayesian credible sets, deserves special mention.

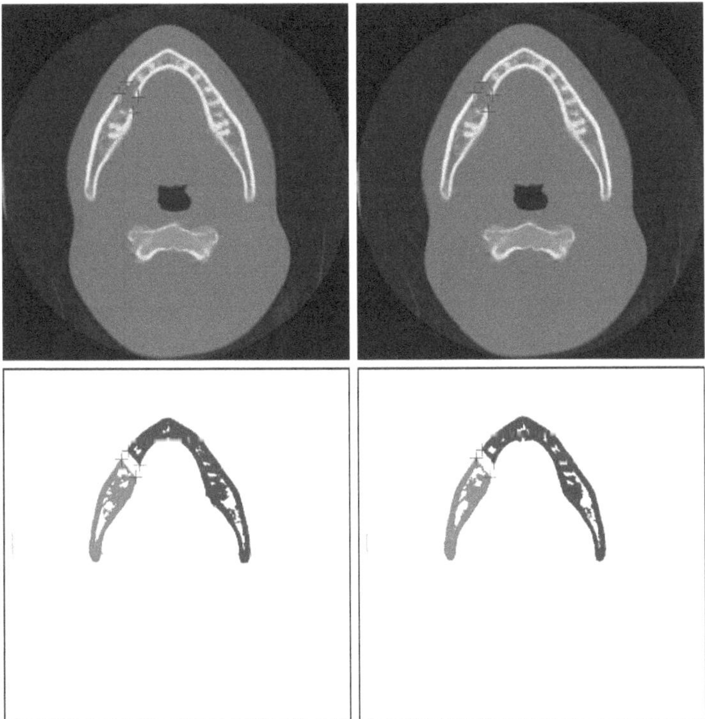

Fig. 6.9 Comparison of stable fracture points detected manually with those detected using the proposed method for two consecutive CT slices of CT dataset-III. The *first row* shows the result of manual fracture point extraction for two consecutive CT slices; the *second row* shows the results of fracture point detection following the Bayesian inference procedure

Table 6.3 Accuracy of Fracture Point Detection

Dataset	(Average Error ± RMS Error)
1	1.88 ± 0.76
2	3.64 ± 1.84
3	3.44 ± 1.23
4	2.42 ± 1.51
5	3.55 ± 3.10

Future work will aim at using bivariate analysis for constructing the highest posterior density credible sets [130]. We also plan to explore the Extended Kalman Filter (EKF) [122] and Particle Filter (PF) [132] in more complex fracture point tracking scenarios involving clutter and highly nonlinear movement of the fracture points. Last, but not least, we plan to extend the proposed methodology for similarly well-displaced fractures at other anatomical sites within the human skeleton, such as those encountered in reconstructive orthopedic surgery.

Chapter 7
Fracture Detection in an MRF-Based Hierarchical Bayesian Framework

7.1 Motivation

The previous chapter discussed the extraction of fracture points and fracture surfaces in the event of a *major fracture* where the bone fragments are well separated. In contrast, the focus of this chapter is on the detection of *hairline fractures* or *minor fractures*. Mandibular fractures are observed to possess certain distinct patterns in X-ray or CT images [2]. In some cases, the fractures are observed to be hairline or minor in nature. By the terms *hairline fracture* or *minor fracture* we refer to those situations where the broken bone fragments are not visibly out of alignment or have incurred very little relative displacement, respectively. The presence of noise makes the detection and subsequent visualization of such types of fractures in X-ray or CT images a very challenging task. In case of a major fracture, i.e., fractures where the broken fragments are clearly displaced relative to each other, surgical intervention is almost mandatory. However, in the case of a hairline fracture or minor fracture, the decision regarding surgical intervention is less clear since the surgeon can rely on natural bone healing for fracture reduction without having to perform reconstructive surgery.

We propose a Markov Random Field (MRF)-based scheme within a hierarchical Bayesian framework for (i) the detection of hairline or minor fractures within the human mandible in the presence of noise and (ii) generation of the reconstructed mandible (i.e., target pattern) upon healing the hairline or minor fractures. In the proposed Bayesian framework, the hypothetical intact mandible is considered to be the *prior*, whereas the input fractured mandible is considered to be the *data*. Estimation of the mode of the *posterior* distribution via Gibbs sampling generates the reconstructed version of the fractured mandible [41]. We assume appropriate statistical distributions on certain variance parameters in the proposed MRF model, thus making the overall Bayesian framework hierarchical. It can be shown that adoption of a hierarchical Bayesian framework has an important advantage of making the output less sensitive to the choice of different hyperparameters used in the MRF model [133]. Finally, the pixel-wise intensity differences between the reconstructed and

A.S. Chowdhury, S.M. Bhandarkar, *Computer Vision-Guided Virtual Craniofacial Surgery*, Advances in Computer Vision and Pattern Recognition,
DOI 10.1007/978-0-85729-296-4_7, © Springer-Verlag London Limited 2011

the fractured mandibles are computed. Substantial intensity differences at certain specific pixel locations mark the occurrence of a fracture.

The target pattern depicts how a jaw with a hairline fracture would appear if allowed to heal naturally without explicit surgical intervention. The target pattern, which is reconstructed *in silico*, has the potential to serve as a potent prognostic tool. By viewing the target pattern, a surgeon can decide if explicit reconstruction via open surgical reduction and fixation is necessary or whether the fractures can be managed by allowing them to heal naturally. In the case of a single major fracture or multiple fractures that are visibly out of alignment, the proposed technique can be used as a smoothing technique at the sites where the opposable bone fragments have been already brought into coarse registration. This would result in the generation of a smooth or continuous 3D model of the reconstructed jaw where the model components corresponding to the individual bone fragments are fused together during free-form solid fabrication. Note that a 3D model is essential for preadaptation of the prostheses needed to stabilize the fractures. The 3D model could also be used to perform the necessary biomechanical analysis to validate the virtual reconstruction of the fractured mandible or craniofacial skeleton along with the affixed prostheses.

From the standpoint of computer vision and pattern recognition research, the problems of hairline fracture detection and target pattern generation are of significant interest. Conventional corner detection techniques for determining points of surface discontinuity, such as the Harris corner detector [134], do not perform well because of the pronounced intensity inhomogeneity and noise present in X-ray and CT images. In the proposed scheme, hairline fracture detection and target pattern generation are achieved simultaneously via an implicit process of image restoration. A visual comparison of an X-ray or CT image of a mandible containing a hairline or minor fracture with that of an unbroken (intact) mandible reveals changes in pixel intensity only in the vicinity of the fracture site. This observation leads to the formulation of an image restoration problem with a *partially unknown local* degradation which is in sharp contrast to the more conventional image restoration problem with a *known global* degradation as outlined by Geman and Geman in their seminal paper [41].

7.2 Chapter Organization

The remainder of the chapter is organized as follows: in Sect. 7.3, we discuss the related research work and highlight our contribution. In Sect. 7.4, we describe the procedure for coarse fracture localization. This section contains three separate subsections. The three Sects. 7.4.1, 7.4.2, and 7.4.3 are respectively devoted to the localization of the mandible in the image, determination of symmetric pixel block pairs as possible fracture sites (where the pixel blocks within each pair lie in opposing halves of the image), and identification of the fracture-containing image half. In Sect. 7.5, we describe the hierarchical Bayesian restoration framework. This section consists of two subsections. In Sect. 7.5.1, we elaborate upon the underlying statistical model, whereas in Sect. 7.5.2, we discuss the formulation of the stochastic degradation matrix. Section 7.6 is devoted to the description and analysis of the experimental results. Section 7.7 concludes the chapter and outlines the directions for future research.

7.3 Related Work and Our Contribution

In this section, we first mention some of the existing applications of the MRF model and the Bayesian restoration paradigm in the area of medical image analysis. For a general review of existing work on fracture detection in X-ray and CT images, the reader is referred to Sect. 6.3 of this monograph. Here, we discuss the theoretical and practical importance of the proposed MRF-based scheme. The two classical applications of the MRF-based paradigm in Bayesian image restoration can be found in the seminal works of Geman and Geman [41] and Besag [135].

Over the past decade, MRF-based techniques have gained popularity for solving various biomedical imaging problems. Some interesting applications include MRF-based image reconstruction for SPECT images by Lee et al. [136], where an MRF is used as a spatial smoothness regularizer; 3D MRF-based volumetric object reconstruction in Magnetic Resonance (MR) images by Choi et al. [137]; multiresolution MRF for tumor detection in mammograms by Chan and Zheng [138]; contextual clustering for analysis of functional MR (fMR) images using an MRF prior by Salli et al. [139]; segmentation of MR brain image data using an MRF and a Gibbs prior by Chen and Metaxas [140]; matching of digital mammograms using Markovian and variational techniques by Richard [141]; a penalized least-squares technique for Borehole Tomography using an MRF and a Gibbs prior by Popa and Zdunek [142]; contour detection of human kidneys using an MRF and active contours by Martin-Fernandez and Alberola-Lopez [143], and reconstruction of MR images from raw Fourier data, where an MRF is used to enforce spatial smoothness, by Raj et al. [144].

To the best of our knowledge, an MRF-based Bayesian hierarchical framework has not been applied previously to the general problem of fracture detection in medical images (X-ray or CT). Figure 7.1 shows the flowchart for detection of hairline or minor fractures using the proposed MRF-based hierarchical Bayesian framework. The proposed scheme takes, as input, a stack of 2D CT image slices of a human mandible with a hairline fracture. As shown in the flowchart (Fig. 7.1), a two-step approach is taken. In the first step, a hairline fracture is localized approximately within a block of pixels by exploiting the (approximate) bilateral symmetry of the human mandible and by using the statistical correlation of the pixel intensities as a measure of intensity mismatch. In the second step, an MRF model-based approach, coupled with Gibbs sampling for the estimation of the posterior mode, is employed on the specific pixel blocks selected in the previous step. As mentioned earlier, the proposed scheme is capable of (i) accurately detecting the fracture, and (ii) generating simultaneously the target pattern.

From a biomedical imaging perspective, the proposed scheme addresses some important clinical issues such as hairline fracture detection and target pattern generation accompanied by a prognosis of fracture healing. The above technique is

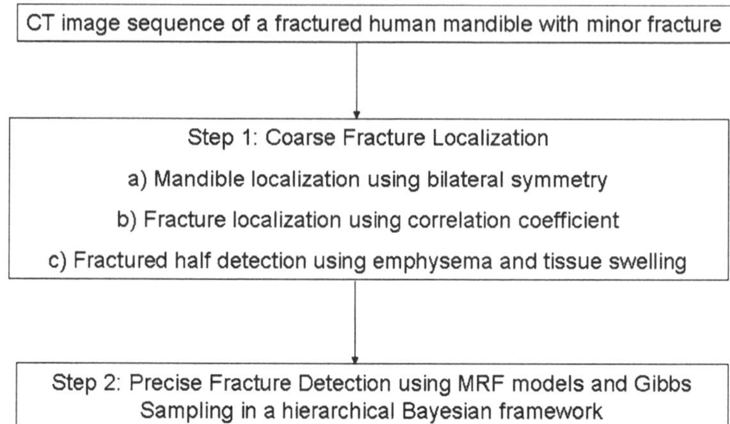

Fig. 7.1 Flowchart for hairline or minor fracture detection

shown to handle input noise in an explicit and efficient manner. The approximate localization of fractures within pixel blocks in the first phase is shown to result in significant computational savings in the second phase. This is so because the MRF modeling and the estimation of posterior mode via Gibbs sampling are restricted only to those pixel blocks in the CT image stack which are known to contain potential fractures. From a theoretical standpoint, the proposed scheme extends the conventional MRF-based paradigm to deal with a *partially unknown local* degradation of image pixel intensities at the fracture site. This is in contrast to the conventional MRF-based paradigm which embodies a *global* and *known* deformation model. The proposed scheme for hairline fracture detection is also designed to perform an implicit restoration of the broken mandible at the fracture sites, thus offering the surgeon a prognostic view of the bone healing process. An initial version of the work described in this chapter can be found in [145].

7.4 Coarse Fracture Localization

The input to the proposed fracture detection scheme is a stack of 2D CT image slices of the human mandible with a hairline fracture. Each 2D CT image slice is assumed to be parallel to the XY plane, whereas the Z axis is assumed to be the axial direction along which the CT image slices are acquired. The bilateral symmetry of the human mandible and the statistical correlation of the pixel intensity values are used for coarse fracture localization. The (approximate) bilateral symmetry of the human mandible is preserved to a great extent in the case of a hairline or minor fracture. The rationale behind using the statistical correlation of pixel or voxel intensity values, computed between pairs of 3D pixel or voxel blocks placed symmetrically in opposing halves of the image, as an indication of the presence of a fracture is that a pair of 3D pixel or voxel blocks in which one block potentially contains a fracture should exhibit a higher intensity mismatch and hence a lower correlation value. In order to ensure that a low correlation value is indeed on account of the presence of a hairline fracture rather than due to existing asymmetry in the CT scan, the position and orientation of the human mandible in the input CT images are first checked. The CT image slices are properly rotated and translated to remove any asymmetry in the existing scans. The CT image stack is divided into a number of 3D pixel or voxel blocks. The fracture localization phase which constitutes the first phase of the proposed two-phase scheme is decomposed into three subphases (see Fig. 7.1) as follows.

7.4.1 Localization of the Mandible

Different anatomical structures within the human body are known to possess different types of symmetry [81]. In the context of our problem, we exploit the (approximate) bilateral symmetry exhibited by the human mandible. As mentioned above, in the case of a hairline or minor fracture, the bilateral symmetry of the mandible is preserved, to a great extent, despite the presence of the fracture. The general equation of a 3D plane (of bilateral symmetry) is given by

$$Ax + By + Cz = D. \tag{7.1}$$

For an axial CT scan of the human mandible, we assumed B and C to be approximately equal to zero and the mandibular cross-section to be approximately centered within each CT image slice of width W. Thus, the equation of the approximate plane of bilateral symmetry reduces to

$$x = W/2. \tag{7.2}$$

For each pixel g_i with coordinates (x, y, z) in the left half of the mandible with a hairline fracture, a bilaterally symmetric pixel g_i^R with coordinates (x^R, y^R, z^R) can be determined as

$$x^R = W - x, \qquad y^R = y, \qquad z^R = z. \tag{7.3}$$

Two heuristics are exploited to reduce the search space for coarse fracture localization. These heuristics along with their justifications (based on domain knowledge) are given below:

1. Since the human mandible is essentially a bony structure, the corresponding pixels or voxels typically exhibit high intensity (i.e., Hounsfield unit) values in the CT images. Consequently, we seek pairs of pixel blocks with high average intensity. This helps to remove pixel blocks containing artifacts and/or large amounts of soft tissue from further consideration.
2. The mandible is typically larger in size compared to other bones in the CT images of the craniofacial skeleton. Since we are primarily interested in detecting mandibular fractures, we perform a second round of filtering by applying the connected component labeling (CCL) algorithm. The CCL algorithm is employed at

the pixel block level rather than at the level of individual pixels. The CCL algorithm is followed by size filtering which serves to eliminate components which span only a small number of pixel blocks.

By using the above heuristics, we essentially retain only a few (say q) pixel blocks which are deemed to contain solely the fractured mandible.

7.4.2 Determination of the Fracture-Containing Symmetric Block Pair(s)

Having localized the mandible in the CT image, the next goal is to localize the fracture within it. This is done by taking a block from the left half of the image, all of whose pixels have x coordinate values such that $0 \leq x \leq W/2$, and a corresponding bilaterally symmetric block in the right half of the image, all of whose pixels have x coordinate values $W/2 \geq x \geq W$, and computing the statistical correlation between the two. The correlation coefficient between a block g, with corresponding pixels g_i, and its bilaterally symmetric counterpart g^R, with corresponding pixels g_i^R, is given by

$$r(g, g^R) = \frac{1}{n-1} \sum_{i=1}^{n} \left(\frac{g_i - \bar{g}}{s_g} \right) \left(\frac{g_i^R - \bar{g}^R}{s_g^R} \right), \tag{7.4}$$

where $\bar{g}$ and $\bar{g}^R$ denote the mean, and s_g and s_g^R denote the standard deviation of the pixels within the blocks g and g^R, respectively.

Having computed a value of $r(g, g^R)$ for each pair of pixel blocks (g, g^R), the pixel block pairs are sorted in increasing order of their $r(g, g^R)$ values. We expect that a hairline fracture will result in some loss of bone material. Consequently, the pixel block within the intact (i.e., unbroken) half of the mandible will contain more pixels with higher intensity values (on account of the presence of more bone material) compared to its bilaterally symmetric counterpart which contains the hairline fracture. Thus, the underlying rationale is that a pair of pixel blocks, in which one of the pixel blocks potentially contains a fracture, should exhibit a higher intensity mismatch and hence a lower correlation value. The user can then choose, based on the correlation values, the best k out of q pixel blocks as sites containing potential hairline fractures. The above technique for coarse fracture localization provides the following two advantages:

1. It achieves computational efficiency by effectively reducing the image size over which the proposed MRF-based scheme coupled with Gibbs sampling is to be applied. Thus, instead of applying the above technique over each CT image slice in its entirety, one needs to do so only over the selected k pixel blocks in each of the slices.
2. It renders the prior shape information in each CT image slice more relevant and more accurate. Instead of determining two quadratic polynomials to describe the

inner contour and outer contour of the entire mandible, we now only need to determine the quadratic polynomials that describe the inner and outer contours of the portion of the mandible that is visible within the selected set of k pixel blocks.

7.4.3 *Identification of the Fracture-Containing Image Half*

After the corresponding pairs of pixel blocks are determined, where the pixel blocks within each pair lie in opposite halves of the CT image slices as determined by the approximate plane of bilateral symmetry, we identify the fracture site using the following two clinical observations:

1. In some CT scans, the fracture sites are marked by the presence of pixel regions with intensity values that are distinctly lower than those of soft tissue and the bone fragments. When the integrity of the soft tissue is violated (due to the impact of the trauma), air can enter the deeper tissue planes and form regions known as *emphysema* that are significantly lower in image intensity than the surrounding soft tissue and bone. The reason emphysema regions appear as dark (low-intensity) spots in the CT scans is due to their low electron density [146, 147].
2. The fracture sites in most CT scans are accompanied by swelling of the soft tissue in the vicinity of the fracture site. When tissue injury occurs, the resulting inflammation increases the capillary permeability in the region. This results in *transudate* and *exudate* formation, which manifests itself in the form of *soft tissue swelling* [146, 147].

We first check for emphysema within the aforementioned localized blocks in the CT image slices. Obviously, the image half which contains the emphysema is designated as the one containing the hairline or minor fracture. In cases, where emphysema is absent, we look for soft tissue swelling. The image half in which the soft tissue swelling is present is deemed to contain the fracture.

7.5 Hierarchical Bayesian Restoration Framework

In this section, we first describe the statistical model formulated to explain the distribution of pixel intensity values within an image. The statistical model is cast within a Bayesian framework. This is followed by the formulation of a stochastic degradation matrix. We prove that in the proposed Bayesian restoration approach the posterior energy function is Gibbsian as defined by Geman and Geman [41]. Although we formulate the model to encompass the entire CT image, we effectively restrict the proposed restoration procedure to the selected localized blocks.

7.5.1 Statistical Model

Let us suppose that we have an image consisting $m \times n$ pixels. Let $p = m \times n$. Based on the formulation detailed in [41], the pixel intensity values in the image can be expressed as

$$g = \Phi(f) + \epsilon, \tag{7.5}$$

where g, f, and ϵ are $p \times 1$ vectors such that g represents the vector of all pixel intensity values in the *observed image*, f represents the vector of pixel intensity values corresponding to the *true image*, and ϵ is zero-mean random Gaussian noise given by

$$\epsilon \sim \mathcal{N}(0, \sigma^2 I_p), \tag{7.6}$$

where $\mathcal{N}(\mu, \sigma^2)$ denotes a Gaussian distribution with mean μ and variance σ^2, and I_p is the pth-order identity matrix. The function $\Phi(\cdot)$ in (7.5) denotes a known degradation (or perturbation) function. Furthermore, we assume that the vector f representing the true pixel intensity values has a known prior distribution. The conditional autoregressive model (CAR) is one of several typical prior distributions that have been used extensively in image processing. The CAR model also ensures the Markovian property of dependence of the intensity value of a pixel on the intensity values of the pixels in its spatial neighborhood [148]. Let τ^2 denote the variance of the prior distribution, and σ^2 the variance of the data model. Therefore,

$$\begin{aligned} p_{\sigma^2}(g|f) &\propto (\sigma^2)^{-p/2} \exp\left\{-\frac{1}{2\sigma^2}\left\|g - \Phi(f)\right\|^2\right\}, \\ p(f \mid \tau^2) &\propto (\tau^2)^{-p/2} \exp\left\{-\frac{1}{2\tau^2} f^T (I_p - \gamma N) f\right\}, \end{aligned} \tag{7.7}$$

where N is the neighborhood matrix given by $N = [n_{ij}]$ where $n_{ii} = 0\ \forall i$ and

$$n_{ij} = \begin{cases} 1 & \text{if } i \text{ and } j \text{ are neighbors,} \\ 0 & \text{otherwise.} \end{cases} \tag{7.8}$$

The value of γ is chosen appropriately to avoid singularity of the matrix $(I_p - \gamma N)$. Also, the prior distributions on σ^2 and τ^2 are chosen as

$$\begin{aligned} p(\sigma^2) &\propto (\sigma^2)^{-(\nu+1)} e^{-\beta/\sigma^2}, \\ p(\tau^2) &\propto (\tau^2)^{-(\kappa+1)} e^{-\delta/\tau^2}. \end{aligned} \tag{7.9}$$

In other words, $\sigma^2 \sim \Gamma^{-1}(\nu, \beta)$ and $\tau^2 \sim \Gamma^{-1}(\kappa, \delta)$, where Γ^{-1} denotes the inverse-gamma distribution. Under this formulation, the posterior distribution of f given the observed data g can be shown to be Gibbsian on account of conjugacy under linear degradation. Before describing the proposed MRF-based scheme in detail, it is important to formulate a precise definition of the term *known degradation* in the present context. In image processing, the term *known degradation* commonly refers to a mathematically known degradation (or blurring) function which is applied to the *entire* true image. The known degradation in conjunction with the (typically additive) noise yields the *observed image*.

For fracture detection, we assume that the image of the fractured mandible is a degraded version of some true (possibly hypothetical) intact mandible. Consequently, the degradation function needs to be formulated in a manner such that if it is applied to the entire true image, i.e., the CT image of the intact mandible, then the resulting image should display a hairline fracture at the desired site while retaining the pixel intensity values of the true image elsewhere. A hairline or minor fracture denotes a loss of bone mass and hence can be modeled as a decrease in the Hounsfield unit (i.e., image intensity) value at the fracture site. Thus, from (7.5), a simple formulation of the degradation function would be

$$g = Af + \epsilon, \tag{7.10}$$

where A is the degradation matrix of order $p \times p$ consisting of nonzero elements only along the diagonal. For the ith pixel,

$$g_i = a_i f_i + \epsilon_i, \tag{7.11}$$

where

$$a_i = \begin{cases} \alpha_i & \text{if } i \text{ is a fracture site,} \\ 1 & \text{otherwise,} \end{cases} \tag{7.12}$$

for some $\alpha_i \in (0, 1)$. The prior distribution of α_i is assumed to be Gaussian:

$$\alpha_i \sim \mathcal{N}(\alpha_{i0}, \eta^2). \tag{7.13}$$

The values of the parameters α_{i0} and η are chosen in such a way that the support of the distribution becomes effectively $(0, 1)$. Later in this section, we provide relevant details on the choice of the value of α_{i0}.

Lemma 7.1 *Under the model characterized by* (7.5)–(7.13), *for a fixed value of* g, *the posterior probability* $p(f|g)$ *is a Gibbs distribution with an associated energy function given by*

$$U(f|g) = \frac{1}{2\sigma^2}\|g - Af\|^2 + \frac{1}{2\tau^2} f^T (I_p - \gamma N) f.$$

For a detailed proof of the above lemma, the interested reader is referred to [41]. As a special case of Lemma 7.1, we formulate the following lemma. Before we formulate the lemma, we introduce the parameter f_{i-} to denote the neighborhood of f_i.

Lemma 7.2 *Based on the MRF formulation in* (7.6) *and* (7.10)–(7.12), *if we assume* $E(f_i|f_{i-}) = \mu(f_{i-})$, *then the posterior distribution of* f_i *given* g_i *and* f_{i-} *can be shown to be* (*see* [130] *for details*)

$$p(f_i|g_i, f_{i-}) \sim \mathcal{N}\left(\frac{\frac{a_i g_i}{\sigma^2} + \frac{\mu(f_{i-})}{\tau^2}}{\frac{a_i^2}{\sigma^2} + \frac{1}{\tau^2}}, \frac{1}{\frac{a_i^2}{\sigma^2} + \frac{1}{\tau^2}} \right).$$

Proof The posterior distribution of $f_i|g_i, f_{i-}$, i.e., $p(f_i|g_i, f_{i-})$ can be expressed as

$$\begin{aligned} p(f_i|g_i, f_{i-}) &\propto \exp\left\{-\frac{1}{2\sigma^2}(g_i - a_i f_i)^2 - \frac{1}{2\tau^2}\left(f_i - \mu(f_{i-})\right)^2\right\} \\ &\propto \exp\left[-\frac{1}{2}\left\{\left(\frac{a_i^2}{\sigma^2} + e\frac{1}{\tau^2}\right) f_i^2 - 2 f_i\left(\frac{a_i g_i}{\sigma^2} + \frac{\mu(f_{i-})}{\tau^2}\right)\right\}\right] \\ &\propto \exp\left\{-\frac{\frac{a_i^2}{\sigma^2} + \frac{1}{\tau^2}}{2}\left(f_i - \frac{\frac{a_i g_i}{\sigma^2} + \frac{\mu(f_{i-})}{\tau^2}}{\frac{a_i^2}{\sigma^2} + \frac{1}{\tau^2}}\right)^2\right\}. \end{aligned}$$ □

In Lemma 7.2 above, it should be noted that $E(f_i|g_i, f_{i-})$ can be seen to be a weighted average of the data and mean of the prior distribution with the weights being functions of the reciprocals of σ^2 and τ^2.

7.5.2 Modeling of the Stochastic Degradation Matrix

A critical issue in the proposed MRF-based formulation described above is an appropriate choice for the values of α_i. A necessary prerequisite for choosing an appropriate value of α_i is some a priori knowledge about the shape of the mandible within the selected pixel blocks in each CT slice. The inner contour and outer contour of the portion of the mandible within the selected set of pixel blocks can each be essentially approximated by a second-degree (i.e., quadratic) polynomial with a distinct set of coefficients. A quadratic polynomial has the general form

$$y = c_0 + c_1 x + c_2 x^2. \tag{7.14}$$

To estimate the coefficients c_0, c_1, and c_2 in (7.14), we need a set of three points, say, $\{(x_1, y_1), (x_2, y_2), (x_3, y_3)\}$, on the inner contour and likewise on the outer contour of the portion of the mandible in the selected set of pixel blocks in each CT image slice comprising the CT image stack. The need to obtain so many data points, i.e., six data points per contour (inner and outer) per CT image slice, can be justified as follows:

1. The inner and outer contours of the mandible, appearing in a given CT image slice, cannot be represented mathematically by a single quadratic polynomial with appropriate translational parameters along the X and Y axes. This is because the curvatures of the inner contour and the outer contour of the mandible are observed to be quite different, resulting in distinct coefficients for the quadratic polynomial in (7.14).
2. Since the spatial resolution of the image stack is coarser along the Z axis (axial direction) compared to the X and Y axes, the inner or outer contour of the mandible in two different slices cannot be approximated mathematically by a single quadratic polynomial. This can also be attributed to the difference in curvatures of an inner or outer contour in two consecutive CT image slices.

Once again, we reemphasize a major advantage of the proposed localization scheme. Fitting a quadratic polynomial to a small portion of the bone surface is more appropriate than fitting it to the entire mandible. Although the entire mandible can be viewed as being roughly parabolic in shape, it is not an exact parabola. A small portion of the mandible, on the other hand, can be represented more accurately by a parabolic contour (which is a quadratic polynomial). Thus, it is more appropriate and convenient to use the quadratic polynomial shape approximation within a small pixel block rather than attempt to derive a complex shape model for the entire mandible. The required data points for the shape approximation are generated automatically. Note that these data points can be from anywhere along the inner (outer) contour of the portion of a mandible delimited by a set of pixel blocks indicating coarse fracture localization. The coefficients of the fitted quadratic polynomial(s) are not particularly sensitive to the choice of the generated points as long as it is ensured that these points lie on the (inner or outer) contour whose equation is being estimated. Once the quadratic polynomial for a contour is determined, a set of points satisfying the polynomial (i.e., a set of points along the fitted contour) is generated. Typically, most of the points within this set have high intensity values, since they correspond to bone pixels, whereas only a few have low intensity values since they correspond to pixels at a potential fracture site. For potential fracture pixels at a site i, on a given contour, the value of α can be ideally assumed to be given by

$$\alpha_i = g_i / \max_i(g_i), \tag{7.15}$$

where $\max_i(g_i)$ represents the maximum of all the observed pixel intensity values along the contour under consideration. Therefore, it is reasonable to assume the mean of α_i $(= \alpha_{i0})$ to be $g_i / \max_i(g_i)$.

Lemma 7.3 *Under the model characterized by* (7.7), (7.9), *and* (7.13), *the full conditional distribution of* α_i *is given by*

$$P(\alpha_i | g_i, f_i) \sim \mathcal{N}\left(\frac{\frac{g_i f_i}{\sigma^2} + \frac{\alpha_{i0}}{\eta^2}}{\frac{f_i^2}{\sigma^2} + \frac{1}{\eta^2}}, \frac{1}{\frac{f_i^2}{\sigma^2} + \frac{1}{\eta^2}} \right).$$

The proof of Lemma 7.3 is very similar to that of Lemma 7.2 given earlier.

Lemma 7.4 *Under the model characterized by* (7.7), (7.9), *and* (7.13), *the full conditional distribution of* σ^2 *is given by*

$$p(\sigma^2 \mid g, f, \alpha) \sim \Gamma^{-1}\left(\frac{p}{2} + \nu, \frac{S + 2\beta}{2} \right),$$

where $S = \|g - Af\|^2$, *and* α *is a vector whose elements are all the* α_i*'s.*

Proof Note that

$$p(\sigma^2, f, g) \propto p_{\sigma^2}(g|f) p(f \mid \tau^2) p(\sigma^2).$$

From (7.7), (7.9), and (7.13) we can write

$$p(\sigma^2 \mid g, f, \alpha) \propto (\sigma^2)^{-\frac{p}{2}-(\nu+1)} \exp\left\{-\frac{S+2\beta}{2\sigma^2}\right\}. \qquad \square$$

Hence the lemma.

Lemma 7.5 *Under the model characterized by* (7.7), (7.9), *and* (7.13), *the full conditional distribution of* τ^2 *is given by*

$$\tau^2 | f, g \sim \Gamma^{-1}\left(\frac{p}{2} + \kappa, \frac{f^T(I_p - \gamma N)f + 2\delta}{2}\right).$$

The proof of the above lemma is similar to that of Lemma 7.4.

It can be noted that all conditional posterior distributions in question have known closed-form expressions. In this situation, we can iteratively draw samples from the posterior distribution using Gibbs sampling. After several iterations, convergence is achieved, and the estimated posterior mode corresponds to the reconstructed version of the target mandible.

7.6 Experimental Results

In this section, we describe the experimental results for the detection of hairline or minor fractures and reconstruction of the target mandible using the proposed two-phase MRF-based scheme, implemented within a hierarchical Bayesian framework. The experiments are performed on different datasets with varying resolution (pixels/mm) and varying fracture position. The fractures are observed to appear typically in 3 to 6 2D slices in each image sequence. Each 2D image slice is 512×512 pixels in size.

In the first phase of the proposed two-phase scheme, we have localized the fracture in blocks by determining the approximate region and the image half in which it appears. The width and the height of a block are sought as inputs from the user via a graphical user interface (GUI). The block thickness is deemed to be the number of 2D slices, in which a fractured mandible appears in a given CT image sequence. Typical values for the width and height of the block are 64×64 pixels and 32×32 pixels. The thickness of a block, i.e., the number of slices in which a fracture appears varies between 3 and 6. However, it is relevant to mention that the proposed scheme is fairly robust to the block dimensions and to the number of block pairs selected as potential hairline or minor fracture sites. For example, from Figs. 7.2–7.3 and Table 7.1 it is evident that the localization works correctly for dataset-I with two different block dimensions given by $64 \times 64 \times 3$ and $32 \times 32 \times 3$. With dimensions of $64 \times 64 \times 3$, 32 pairs of blocks are examined. After the two heuristics based on mandible size and bone pixel intensity are applied (see Sect. 7.4.1), only 8 out of 32 pairs of blocks are observed to qualify as potential hairline or minor fracture sites. These are then arranged in order of increasing value of the correlation coefficient.

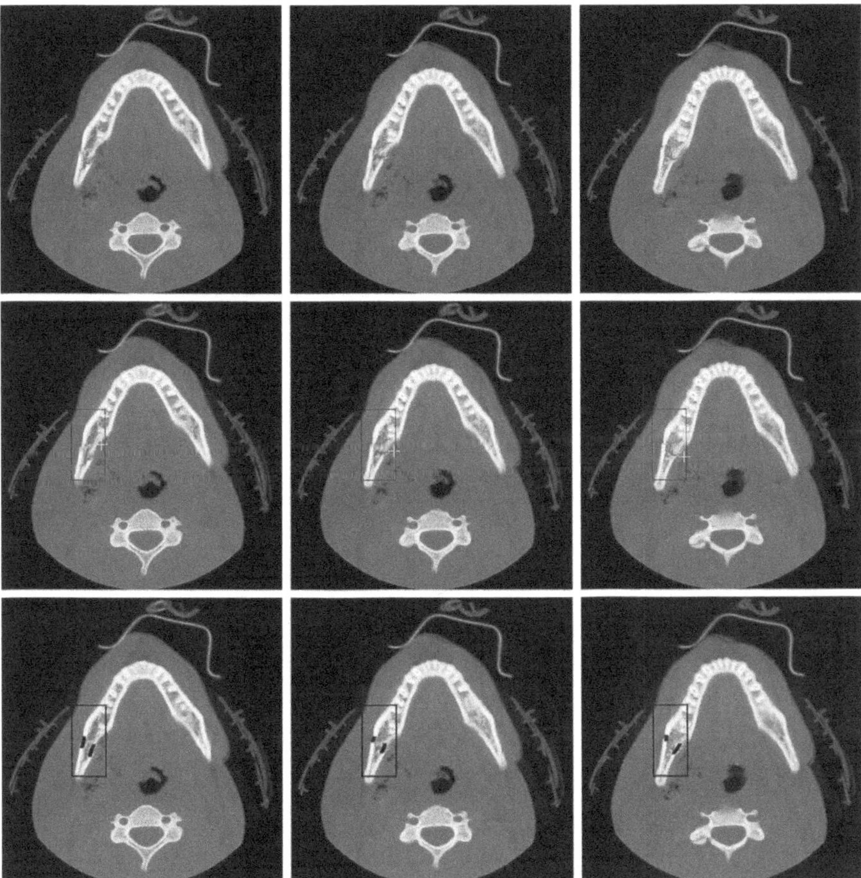

Fig. 7.2 Fracture detection results for dataset-I. The *first* (*topmost*) *row* shows the input CT image sequence. The *second row* and *third row* show respectively the results of fracture localization and precise fracture detection. The pixel block size is 64 × 64 × 3, and two symmetrical pixel blocks are selected via correlation. Additionally, the *centers of white crosses in the second row* mark the detection of *emphysema*

Finally, 2 out of these 8 block pairs are chosen as potential hairline or minor fracture sites (see Sect. 7.4.2). For the same dataset, with dimensions of 32 × 32 × 3, only 13 out of possible 128 block pairs are retained using the aforementioned heuristics based on mandible size and bone pixel intensity. Eventually, 4 out of 13 block pairs are chosen as potential hairline or minor fracture sites based on the correlation coefficient values. Table 7.1 details the experimental results for five sample datasets with two different block dimensions. Table 7.1 also shows the number of selected block pairs based on the correlation coefficient values in each case and the typical values of the correlation coefficient for blocks that potentially contain hairline or minor fractures.

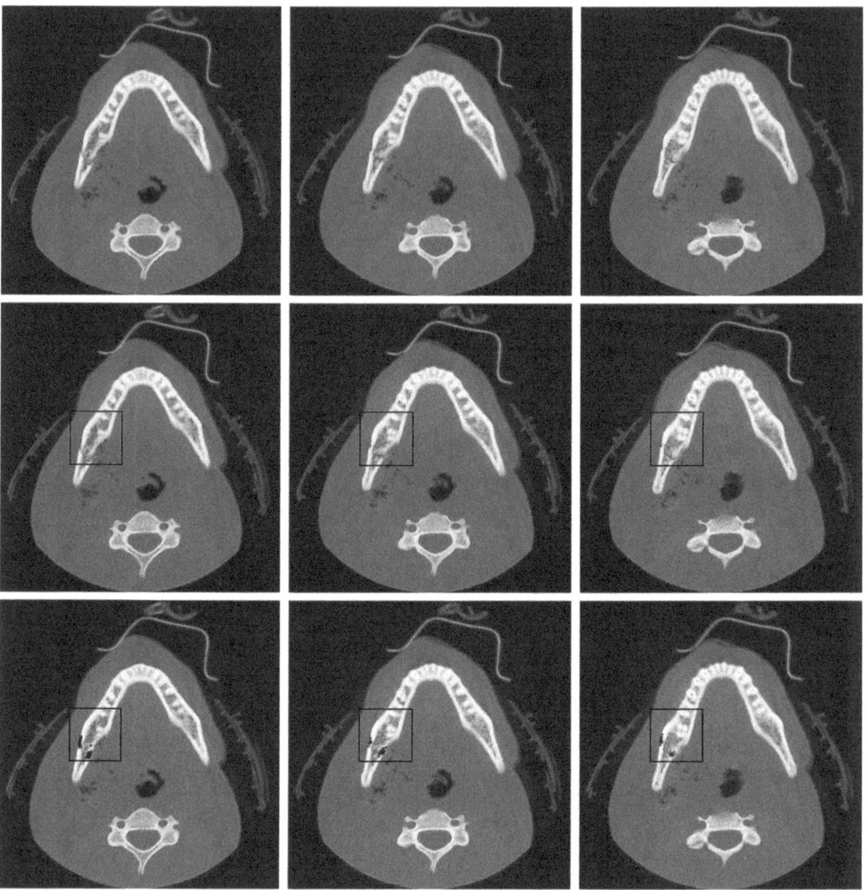

Fig. 7.3 Fracture detection results for dataset-I. The *first* (*topmost*) *row* shows the input CT image sequence. The *second row* and *third row* show respectively the results of fracture localization and precise fracture detection. The pixel block size is $32 \times 32 \times 3$, and four symmetrical pixel blocks are selected via correlation

Table 7.1 Results of fracture localization in five sample datasets

Dataset	Block Size	Potential Block Pairs	Selected Block Pairs	Correlation Coeff.
1	$64 \times 64 \times 3$	8	2	0.022, 0.038
	$32 \times 32 \times 3$	13	4	0.007, 0.068, 0.109, 0.153
2	$32 \times 32 \times 3$	15	2	0.012, 0.036
3	$32 \times 32 \times 3$	11	2	0.03, 0.16
	$32 \times 32 \times 3$	11	3	0.03, 0.16, 0.23
4	$32 \times 32 \times 4$	8	4	0.002, 0.028, 0.087, 0.144
5	$32 \times 32 \times 3$	9	2	0.029, 0.101

Table 7.2 Detection of the fractured half of the mandible in five sample datasets

Dataset	Emphysema	Tissue Swell. (pix. dist.)	Frac. Half
1	Left	–	Left
2	–	left: 65, right: 54	Left
3	Left	–	Left
4	–	left: 36, right: 79	Right
5	–	left: 44, right: 76	Right

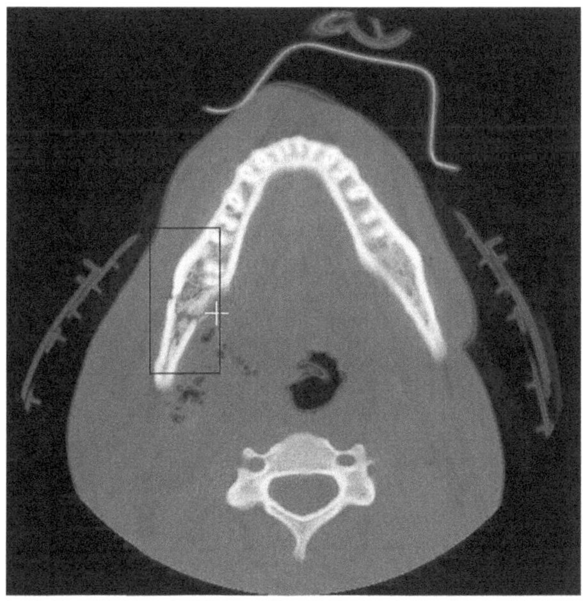

Fig. 7.4 Enlarged version of the first slice in Fig. 7.2 to better illustrate the detection of *emphysema*, marked by the *centers of the white crosses*

Next, we discuss the determination of the image half containing the potential fracture (see Sect. 7.4.3). Table 7.2 demonstrates the detection of emphysema and soft tissue swelling in two and three of the sample datasets, respectively. The detection of emphysema is marked by the presence of white crosses in Fig. 7.2. A clearer illustration of the detection of emphysema is provided in Fig. 7.4, where an enlarged version of the first slice in Fig. 7.2 is shown. Note that we have marked just one particular pixel site to denote the occurrence of emphysema in both Figs. 7.2 and 7.4. In reality, there exist quite a few such emphysema pixels. Obviously, the CT image half in which emphysema is detected is designated as the one containing fracture site. Swelling of soft tissue is another anatomical observation that is associated with a potential hairline fracture. A clearer illustration of the swelling of soft tissue is provided in Fig. 7.8. The inter-pixel distance is employed as a quantitative measure to detect the swelling of soft tissue. The average of inter-pixel distances between the outer soft tissue boundary and the center of each block within a symmetric block pair (in which a potential fracture is coarsely localized via correlation) is computed.

Table 7.3 Coefficients of the quadratic polynomial fit for the outer and inner contours for three different CT image slices in dataset-I

Quad. Poly. Coeffs.	Slice 1		Slice 2		Slice 3	
$(c_0 + c_1x + c_2x^2)$	Outer	Inner	Outer	Inner	Outer	Inner
c_0	−11344	6808	8798	5228.7	−177200	−107.19
c_1	162	75.7	−113.2	67.8	2380	5.79
c_2	−1	2	4	2	−10	−0.02

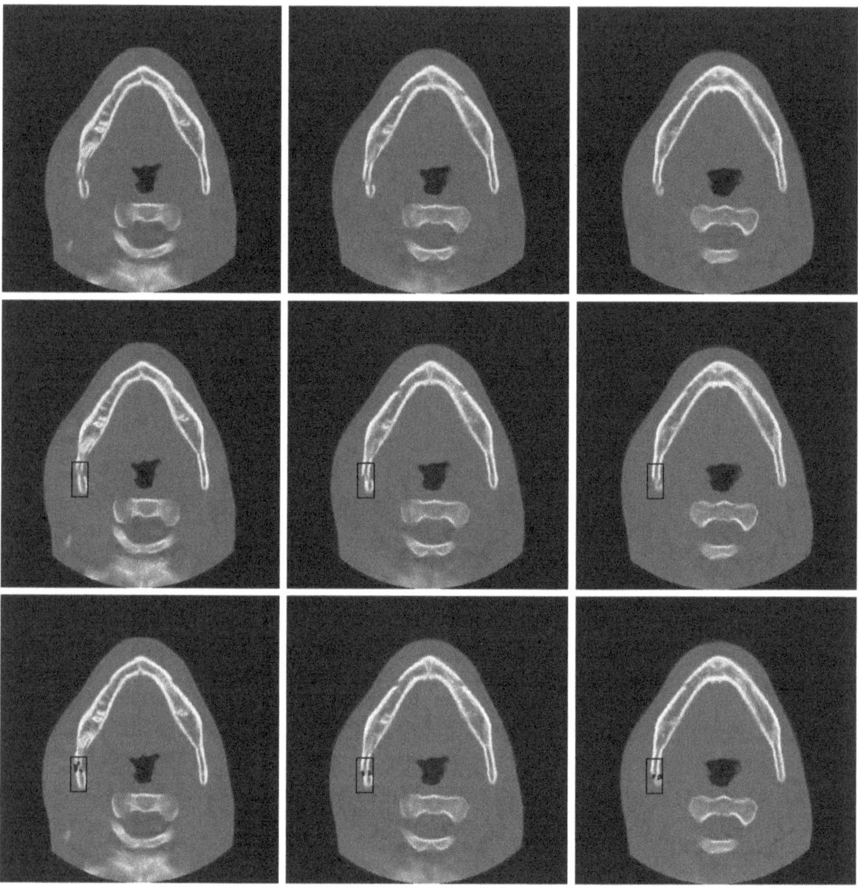

Fig. 7.5 Fracture detection results for dataset-II. The *first* (*topmost*) *row* shows the input CT image sequence. The *second row* and *third row* show respectively the results of fracture localization and precise fracture detection

Note that each block within a symmetric block pair lies within a half of an image slice. The image half in which the average inter-pixel distance is higher than a prespecified threshold, indicates the presence of soft tissue swelling and hence the

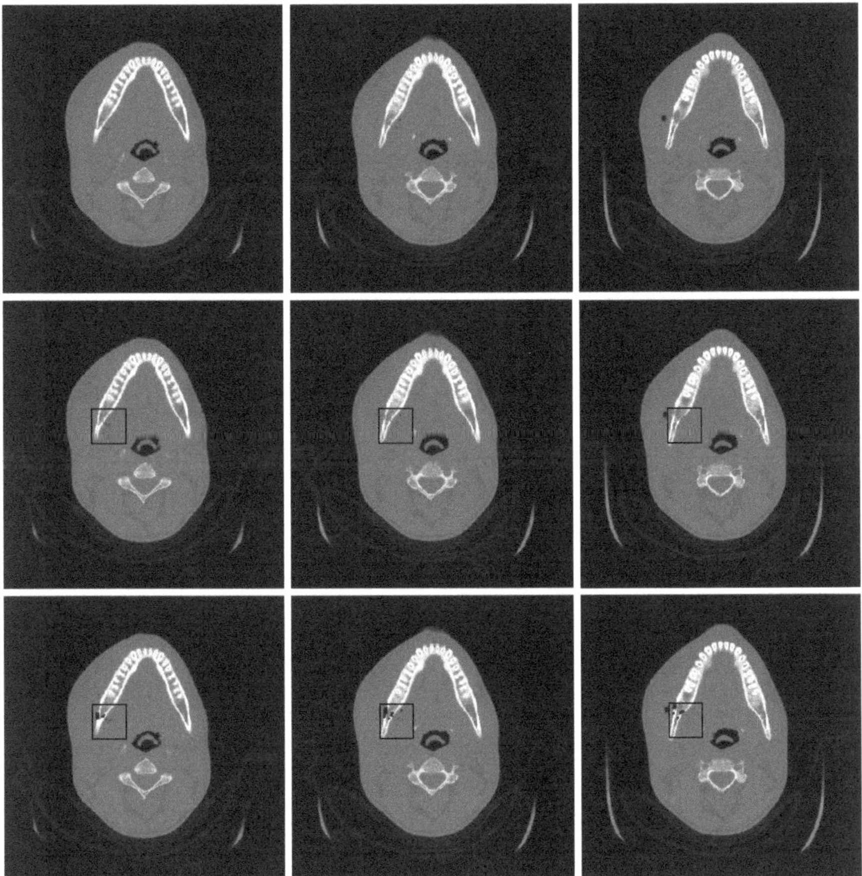

Fig. 7.6 Fracture detection results for dataset-III. The *first* (*topmost*) *row* shows the input CT image sequence. The *second row* and *third row* show respectively the results of fracture localization and precise fracture detection

fracture site. In this manner, at the end of the first phase, we identify only a few blocks within one half of the image that could potentially contain the hairline or minor fracture.

In order to estimate the stochastic degradation matrix representing a fractured mandible (that is coarsely localized within a block or few block(s)), a quadratic polynomial fitting technique is employed (see Sect. 7.5.2). In Table 7.3, we show the typical values of the three coefficients of a quadratic polynomial, shown in (7.14), to approximate the inner and outer mandibular contours for a sample CT dataset. From Table 7.3, it is quite clear that for a given image slice, the outer and inner contours of a jaw cannot be modeled by two (approximately) parallel quadratic polynomials since all the three coefficients of the inner and outer contours are significantly different. Thus, six data points are required per CT image slice, i.e., three data points for the inner contour and three data points for the outer contour. Table 7.3 also demon-

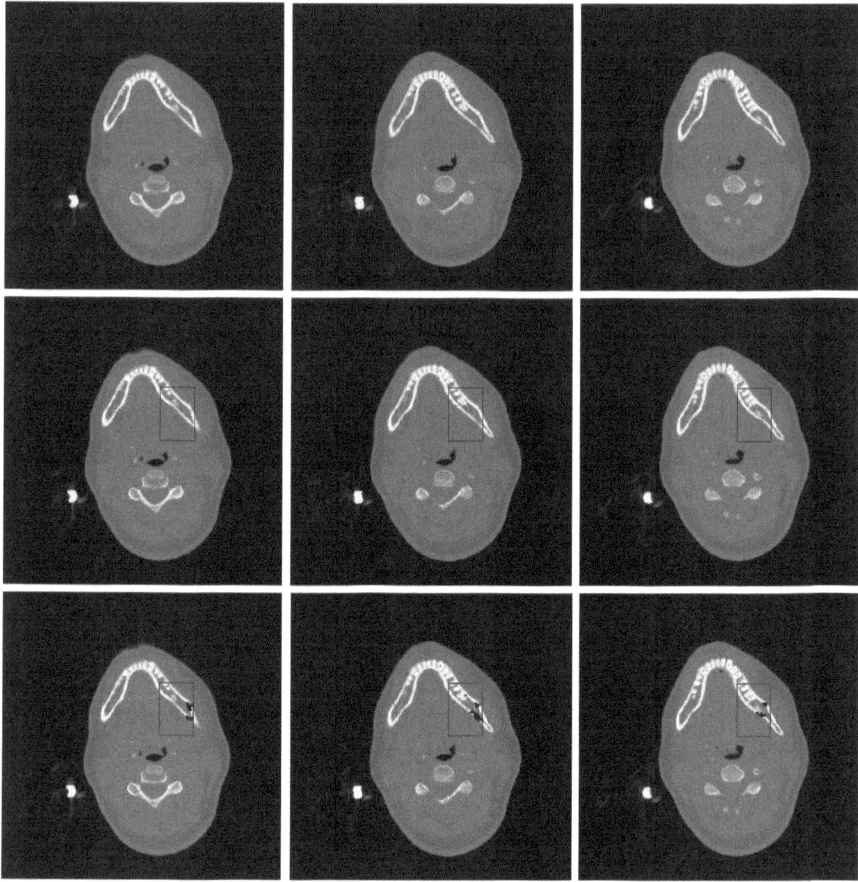

Fig. 7.7 Fracture detection results for dataset-IV. The *first* (*topmost*) *row* shows the input CT image sequence. The *second row* and *third row* show respectively the results of fracture localization and precise fracture detection

strates that a single quadratic polynomial cannot be used to approximate either the outer or inner mandibular contour in *all* of the fracture-containing CT image slices. Thus, it is necessary to identify six distinct points for *each* 2D CT image slice that is deemed to potentially contain a hairline or minor fracture. These points are generated automatically without the need for any user intervention. Domain knowledge about possible fracture point intensity values is exploited in order to estimate the degradation matrix. Thus, using (7.15), we assign a value of 1 to a_i if α_i is in the range [0.85, 1]; otherwise, we assign a_i to be the mean of α_i. For the MRF-based formulation, a first-order neighborhood is selected. As far as the statistical parameters are concerned, we choose the shape and scale of the inverse gamma distribution for τ^2 to be 3.0 and 1.0 and for σ^2 to be 3.0 and 0.5, respectively. We assume that 100 iterations are adequate to ensure convergence of the Gibbs sampling pro-

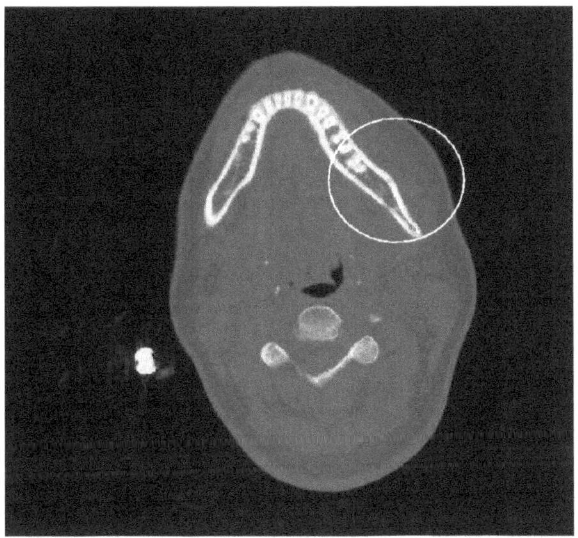

Fig. 7.8 Enlarged version of the second slice in Fig. 7.7. Tissue swelling near the fracture site is illustrated with a *white circle*

cedure. In fact, visual inspection of the reconstructed output indicated no noticeable improvement if the number of iterations was increased beyond 100.

The completion of each phase of the proposed two-phase scheme takes about 2–3 minutes on a 1.73-GHz Intel Pentium-M© processor. It is relevant to discuss here why we have opted for a partial 3D scheme for the purpose of fracture detection, instead of a scheme that is strictly 3D. The localization procedure is essentially a 3D scheme as the correlation is computed over a single 3D block instead of multiple 2D blocks in individual 2D slices. The estimation of the degradation matrix calls for prior fitting of polynomial curves to the inner and outer mandibular contours. It is visually intuitive to fit a quadratic polynomial to portions of these contours within the localized block(s) in the individual 2D CT image slices. Thus, as mentioned earlier, we can circumvent the computational complexity of fitting more complex 3D shape models to the entire 3D mandibular surface. Furthermore, since the number of image slices within a CT image stack in which a fracture appears is often few (typically 3 to 6), a complete 3D scheme would not have resulted in significant performance improvement in terms of the overall localization accuracy or execution time.

We show here the images depicting the results of the fracture detection procedure for seven sample datasets (see Figs. 7.2, 7.3, 7.5, 7.6, 7.7, 7.9, 7.10, 7.11). The first (topmost) row in each of these figures depicts successive slices from a CT image sequence of a mandible with a minor or hairline fracture. The second row in each of these figures illustrates the results of the coarse fracture localization procedure in the corresponding CT image slices. Figures 7.2 and 7.3 depict the results of the fracture localization procedure performed using pixel blocks of two different dimensions on the same dataset (dataset-I). Consequently, the numbers of potential blocks selected, in each of these two cases, in order to localize the same fracture are also different. For all the above seven CT image datasets, the localized fractures

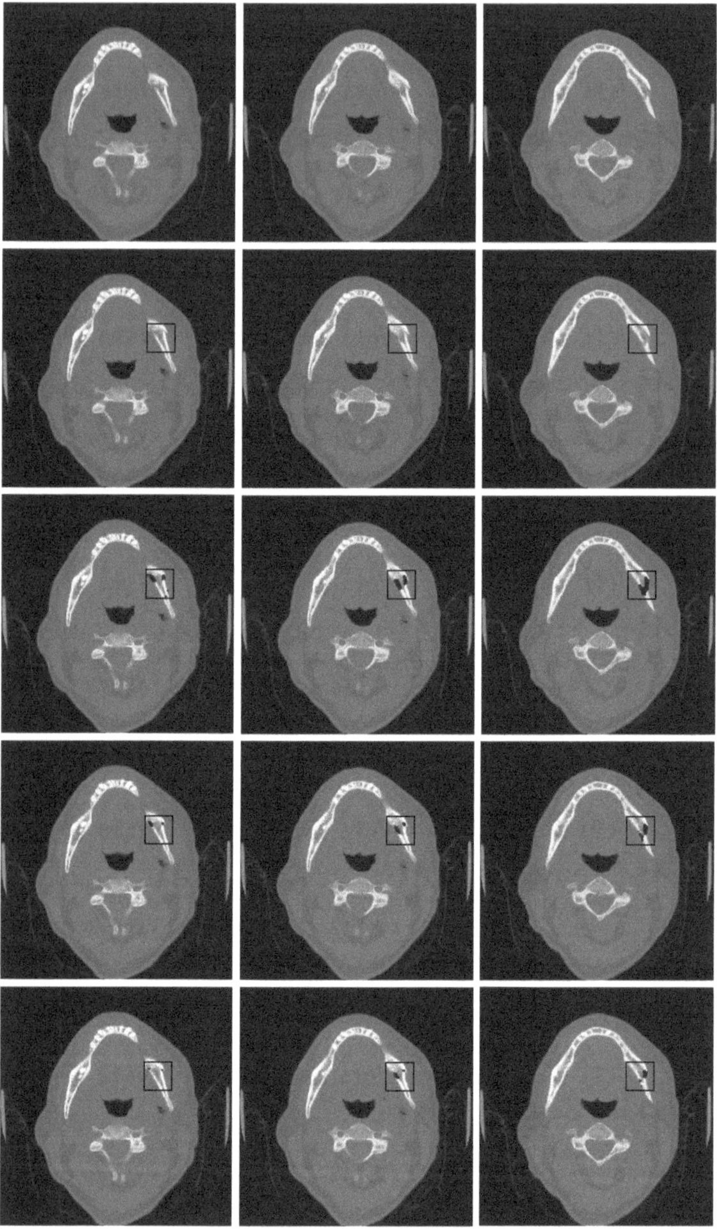

Fig. 7.9 Fracture detection results for dataset-V. The *first* (*topmost*) *row* shows the input CT image sequence. The *second row* shows the localization of the fracture. The *third*, *fourth*, and *fifth rows* show the precise detection and visualization of the fracture for successively increasing values of the threshold. The threshold value is a measure of the difference in intensity between the input data and the reconstructed data

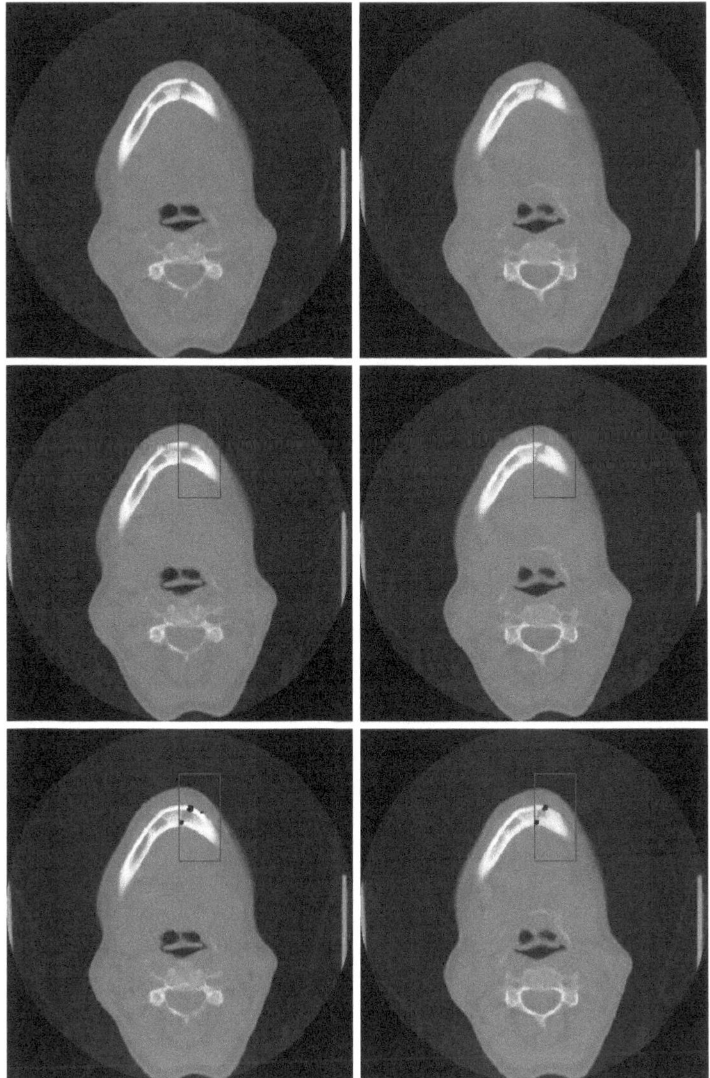

Fig. 7.10 Fracture detection results for dataset-VI. The *first* (*topmost*) *row* shows the input CT image sequence. The *second row* and *third row* show respectively the results of fracture localization and precise fracture detection

are highlighted by the surrounding black boxes at the fracture sites. The third row in each of these figures shows the results of the precise fracture detection and visualization procedures using MRF-based modeling and Gibbs sampling. Note that whereas the original intensity values at the pixel sites of the fracture are low (due to loss of bone material), the reconstructed (restored) intensity values at these sites are high (corresponding to the pixel intensities of bone material) on account of es-

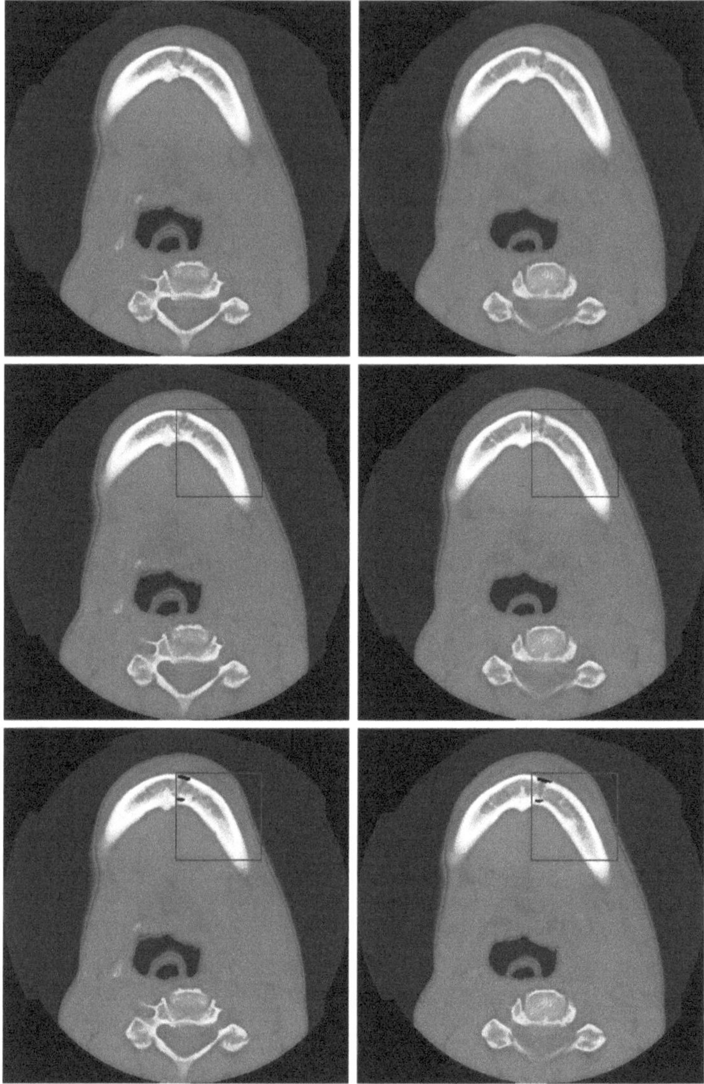

Fig. 7.11 Fracture detection results for dataset-VII. The *first* (*topmost*) *row* shows the input CT image sequence. The *second row* and *third row* show respectively the results of fracture localization and precise fracture detection

timation of the posterior mode via repetitive Gibbs sampling. The pixels exhibiting large intensity differences between the reconstructed and the fractured mandible are highlighted using the color black for the purpose of visualization of the hairline or minor fracture.

The detection of the hairline or minor fractures was validated by experienced surgeons and radiologists. In this context, we would like to discuss the choice of

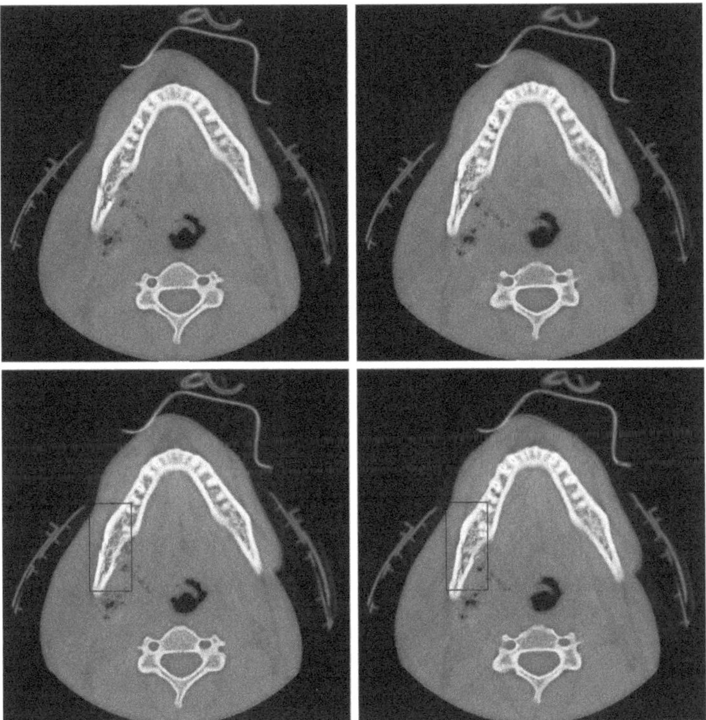

Fig. 7.12 Target pattern generation for dataset-I. The *first* (*top*) *row* shows CT image slices of the fractured jaw and the *second* (*bottom*) *row* shows the corresponding CT image slices of the reconstructed jaw

a threshold value for the difference in intensity between the input data and the reconstructed data that can be used to visualize a fracture. If the user selects a high threshold value (i.e., a large difference in intensity between the input data and the reconstructed data), the final fracture appearance will be quite restricted. In contrast, if the user selects a lower value for this threshold, i.e., a small difference in intensity between the input data and the reconstructed data), the fracture at the proper locations will be displayed more prominently with a chance of picking up some spurious appearances (due to spatial spread). This fact is well illustrated by Fig. 7.9, where the results of a monotonically increasing threshold value are depicted from the third row through the fifth row. This procedure for adjusting the threshold can be viewed as turning a practical knob for controlling or tuning the extent of visualization (i.e., prominence) of the hairline or minor fractures.

We end this section with a brief discussion on the target pattern generation procedure. Figures 7.12, 7.13, and 7.14 depict the generated target patterns for three different datasets. The first row in each of these figures depicts the fractured mandible, whereas the second row illustrates the *in silico* reconstruction of the fractured mandible, generated using the proposed MRF-based approach. It is quite evident that the reconstructed mandibles in Figs. 7.12 and 7.13 exhibit relatively smooth

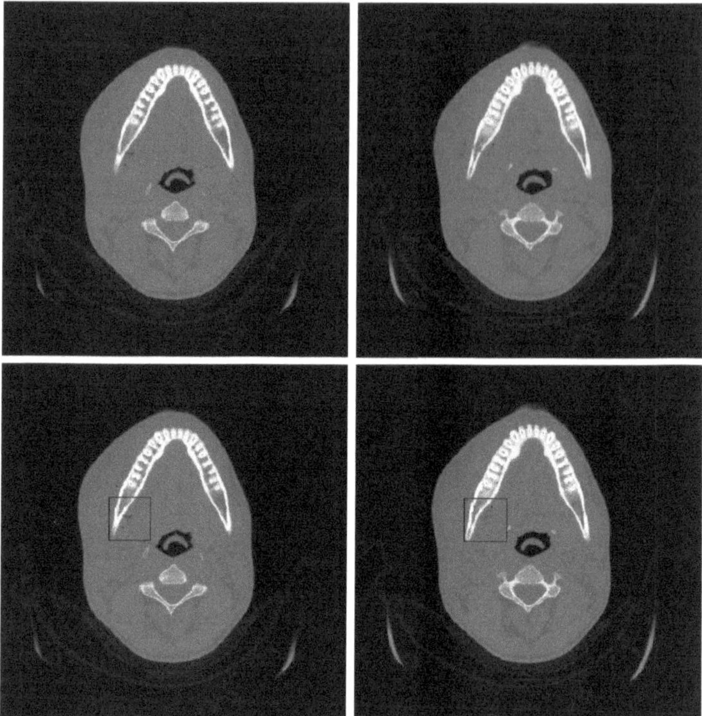

Fig. 7.13 Target pattern generation for dataset-III. The *first* (*top*) *row* shows CT image slices of the fractured jaw, and the *second* (*bottom*) *row* shows the corresponding CT image slices of the reconstructed jaw.

inner and outer contours, which, in turn, indicates that natural bone healing (i.e., absence of surgical intervention) could be opted for in such cases. However, the reconstructed mandible in Fig. 7.14 exhibits inner and outer contours that are not smooth, suggesting thereby that surgical intervention may be more appropriate in this case.

7.7 Conclusion and Future Work

In this chapter, we presented a novel two-phase scheme for detection of hairline or minor fractures in the human mandible and simultaneous generation of the target pattern or reconstructed mandible upon fracture healing. The fracture detection scheme is robust to the presence of noise and intensity inhomogeneity in the CT images. The reconstructed mandible is viewed as a target pattern which can assist a surgeon in determining whether manual surgical intervention is necessary or whether natural bone healing is adequate.

In the first phase of the proposed two-phase approach, the hairline or minor fractures are localized within the pixel blocks of a given size by analyzing all the image

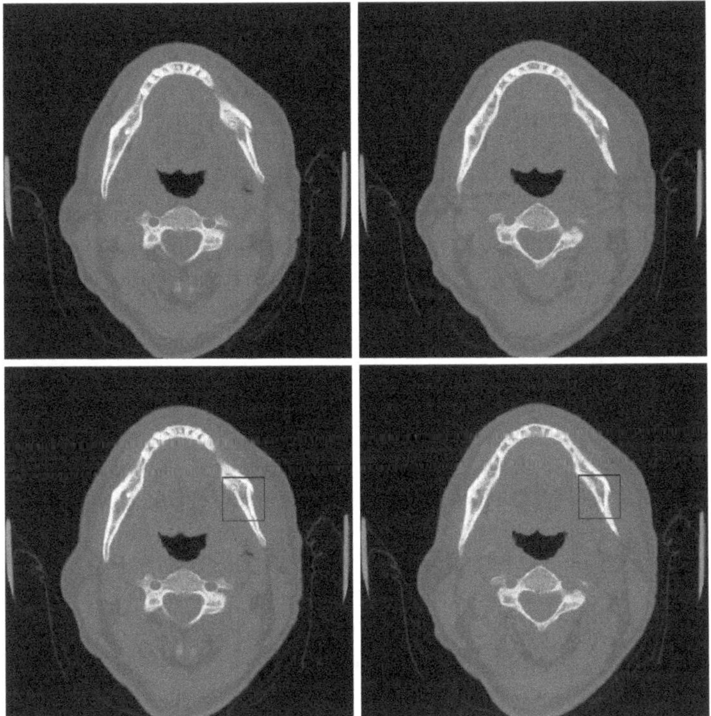

Fig. 7.14 Target pattern generation for dataset-V. The *first* (*top*) *row* shows CT image slices of the fractured jaw, and the *second* (*bottom*) *row* shows the corresponding CT image slices of the reconstructed jaw

slices in the CT image stack. The CT image analysis exploits the (approximate) bilateral symmetry of the human mandible and uses the statistical correlation coefficient as a measure of intensity mismatch. The CT image half in which a fracture appears is determined by exploiting domain knowledge that includes the presence of *emphysema* and *soft tissue swelling*. In each of the aforementioned pixel blocks, an MRF-based approach for detection of hairline or minor fractures is employed. The proposed MRF-based technique is observed to outperform existing conventional techniques based on corner detection or discontinuity detection in the image intensity surface. The hairline fracture detection scheme, in addition to its obvious diagnostic utility, has the potential to be used as a prognostic tool as well. Since the implicit reconstruction procedure embedded within the proposed MRF-based technique is designed to mimic the natural bone healing process in the absence of surgical intervention, the proposed scheme has clear prognostic utility.

In addition to its obvious clinical significance, the problem of hairline fracture detection also possesses certain noteworthy aspects of theoretical interest from the perspective of computer vision and pattern recognition research. This is primarily because we are faced with the challenging task of modeling a *spatially localized* degradation resulting from a mathematically *unknown* degradation function. Thus, we first computed the degradation matrix from the input data by fitting quadratic polynomial functions to the inner and outer contours of the mandible. This was followed by the application of the Gibbs sampling procedure for the estimation of the mean of the posterior distribution. In the current implementation, the degradation matrix A is modeled as a stochastic entity, by imposing a normal distribution on the α values. Additionally, we used the inverse-gamma distribution for both, the variance of the prior distribution τ^2 and the variance of the data model σ^2, in order to conform to the hierarchical Bayesian estimation paradigm.

A potential direction for future research entails automatic identification of the set of 2D CT image slices containing the fractured mandible from a larger set of CT images. Note that a typical CT image sequence is an aggregation of 2D image slices where only some of the image slices contain the fractured mandible. We also intend to explore the utility of the present MRF-based approach as a smoothing tool. We can potentially employ the proposed scheme as a smoothing procedure on instances of well-displaced fractures that have been coarsely registered [54]. This would allow us to generate a more realistic 3D model of the reconstructed mandible resulting in a more accurate analysis of its biomechanical stability. From a statistical perspective, we plan to investigate the effects of (a) a higher-order neighborhood (such as a second-order neighborhood) for the proposed MRF model, (b) an alternative to the CAR model, such as the simultaneous autoregressive (SAR) model [40], and (c) an objective assumption on the prior distribution of the variance parameters which would make the problem formulation more general but also computationally more challenging [39].

Chapter 8
Fracture Detection Using Max-Flow Min-Cut

8.1 Motivation

In this chapter, we propose an alternative technique for detection and localization of mandibular fractures using the concepts underlying network flow. Mandibular fractures exhibit certain distinct patterns in X-ray or CT images, as described in [2]. As mentioned earlier in this monograph, the fractures could be either (a) *hairline* or *minor*, denoting situations where the broken bone fragments are not visibly out of alignment or have incurred very little relative displacement, or (b) *major*, denoting situations where the broken fragments are clearly displaced relative to each other. In the previous chapter, we modeled a minor or hairline fracture as a stochastic degradation of a hypothetical intact mandible. Here, we model a fracture as a discontinuity or *cut* in the flow of intensities between two designated points, termed as the *source* and *sink* in a directed graph or flow network. A fracture is detected by determining a minimum cut in the flow network using the well-known Maximum-Flow Minimum-Cut (Max-Flow Min-Cut) algorithm by Ford and Fulkerson [36]. This approach for identification and localization of fractures is shown to yield more promising results in the case of minor fractures while requiring very little preprocessing of the input image data. We first model a sequence of 2D CT image slices as a collection of independent 2D directed graphs and execute the max-flow min-cut algorithm on each such directed graph. Later, we model the sequence of 2D CT image slices containing a fractured mandible as one complete 3D directed graph and run the same max-flow min-cut algorithm on it.

8.2 Chapter Organization

The remainder of this chapter is organized as follows: in Sect. 8.3, we discuss the related work and highlight our contribution. In Sect. 8.4, we describe the procedure for fracture detection in individual 2D CT image slices. Section 8.4 contains two separate subsections. In Sect. 8.4.1, the construction of the flow network is detailed,

A.S. Chowdhury, S.M. Bhandarkar, *Computer Vision-Guided Virtual Craniofacial Surgery*, Advances in Computer Vision and Pattern Recognition,
DOI 10.1007/978-0-85729-296-4_8,

whereas in Sect. 8.4.2, the mathematical modeling of fracture detection as a max-flow min-cut problem is justified. The analysis presented in Sect. 8.4 for a single 2D CT image slice and is extended in Sect. 8.5 for a 3D CT image stack. Section 8.5 contains two subsections. Section 8.5.1 discusses the construction of the 3D flow network, whereas Sect. 8.5.2 justifies intuitively the underlying 3D network flow model. Section 8.6 is devoted to the presentation and analysis of experimental results. Finally, in Sect. 8.7, the chapter is concluded with an outline of future research directions.

8.3 Related Work and Our Contribution

In this section, we first review previous applications of graph cuts in computer vision with special emphasis on medical image analysis. Minimization of an energy function via graph cuts was first introduced by Boykov et al. [149] in the context of image segmentation. Boykov and Jolly [150] have presented experimental results of a graph cut-based segmentation algorithm on abdominal CT images in 2D and 3D. The network flow capacity function of Boykov and Jolly [150] is based on pixel intensity values and interpixel distance values. In their work, Freedman and Zhang [152] have introduced shape-based priors to extend the graph cut-based segmentation framework proposed by Boykov and Jolly [150]. Xu et al. [151] have enhanced the performance of graph cut-based image segmentation algorithms by the incorporation of active contour models. In their work on CT coronary visualization, Funka-Lea et al. [153] have used graph cuts for automatic heart isolation. Similarly, Song et al. [154] have proposed an adaptive version of the graph cut algorithm for brain MRI segmentation that incorporates a tissue-based prior. It is to be noted that most researchers have employed the framework of Boykov and Jolly [150] with different forms for the energy function. For a more recent as well as comprehensive coverage on graph cuts for multidimensional image segmentation, the reader is referred to another seminal paper by the same authors [155]. For existing work on fracture detection in X-ray or CT images, the reader should revisit Sect. 6.3 of this monograph.

In mandibular fracture detection, the focus is on detecting and localizing discontinuities or cuts on the boundaries of a fractured mandible rather than on image segmentation per se. Our principal contribution lies in the innovative mathematical modeling of the mandibular fracture detection and localization problem as a max-flow min-cut problem in a flow network. Given a 2D CT image slice, the two condyles of the human mandible are deemed to be a natural choice for the source and the sink vertices in a flow network. In an unbroken mandible, the value of the maximum flow between the two condyles is expected to be very high. In a fractured mandible, one expects a significant drop in the value of the maximum flow. The location of the minimum cut is deemed to mark the occurrence of a fracture, and the magnitude of the flow is deemed to provide an indication of the extent of the fracture. To the best of our knowledge, the approach based on determination of maximum-flow minimum-cut in a flow network has not been employed previously for fracture detection and localization in general, and certainly not for the detection and localization of mandibular fractures.

8.4 Max-Flow Min-Cut in a 2D Flow Network

In this section, we first discuss the construction of the flow network representation for a 2D CT slice with suitable choices for the vertices, edges, and capacity functions for the computation of the edge weights. We then justify our claim that the fracture detection and localization problem is equivalent to that of identification and localization of a minimum cut in an appropriately constructed flow network.

8.4.1 Construction of the 2D Flow Network

In their formulation of a flow network for image segmentation, Boykov and Jolly [150] choose all the pixels in an image as the vertices of the flow network and establish edge connections between a pixel and its 8-neighbors. Since our problem is one of fracture detection and not image segmentation per se, we take a different approach to the construction of the flow network $G = (V, E)$. It is noticed that a typical minor fracture is visible on and in the vicinity of the bone contours. Even in the case of a major fracture, a break in the bone contours is prominently visible. This motivates us to select the set of boundary pixels P on the two mandibular contours (i.e., the inner contour and outer contour) as the vertices of the proposed flow network. Let the outer contour and the inner contour be denoted by q and r, respectively. The first and last vertices of the outer contour are denoted by q_f and q_l, respectively, and those of the inner contour by r_f and r_l, respectively.

We identify the two condyles which are anatomical landmark points at the two opposite extremities of the mandible as natural choices for the source vertex s and the sink vertex t of the flow network. The vertex set V is given by $V = P \cup \{s, t\}$. Thus, each pixel on the outer and inner contours of the mandible is a vertex of the flow network. We construct the *tangential* edges T and the *normal* edges N of the flow network as follows. For each pixel on the inner and outer mandibular contours, we create edges linking the pixel with its immediately preceding pixel and immediately succeeding pixel along the same contour. These constitute the T edges of the flow network. On the other hand, an N edge is established between each pair of pixels on opposing contours (i.e., one pixel lies on the inner contour, and the other lies on the outer contour) such that the resulting edge is normal (or approximately normal) to a T edge containing one of the pixels. In addition, the first boundary pixel of the outer contour q_f and that of the inner contour r_f are each attached to the source vertex s, and the last boundary pixel of the outer contour q_l and that of the inner contour r_l are each attached to the sink vertex t. Therefore,

$$E = T \cup N \cup \{(q_f, s), (r_f, s), (q_l, t), (r_l, t)\}.$$

The rationale behind having tangential and normal edges is guided by the geometry of the mandible as well as the geometry of the fracture pattern. A fracture can occur along the two mandibular contours (covered by tangential edges) or across these contours (covered by normal edges). Let j and k be any two consecutive points on one of the mandibular contours with coordinates (x_j, y_j) and (x_k, y_k), respectively. Then the equation of the line that is normal to the contour at point j is given by

$$(x_k - x_j)x + (y_k - y_j)y + \big(x_j(x_j - x_k) + y_j(y_j - y_k)\big) = 0. \tag{8.1}$$

In order to be a normal neighbor to the point j, a point on the opposing contour should ideally satisfy (8.1). However, primarily due to sampling error, it is not always possible to find the exact normal neighbor. So, we compute the distance d_{jm} of a set of competing candidate points m having coordinates (m_x, m_y) and choose the one which yields the minimum value of d_{jm}. From basic coordinate geometry, we obtain

$$d_{jm} = \frac{Am_x + Bm_y + C}{\sqrt{A^2 + B^2}}, \tag{8.2}$$

where $A = (x_k - x_j)$, $B = (y_k - y_j)$, and $C = (x_j(x_j - x_k) + y_j(y_j - y_k))$. We choose a very simple capacity function, with pixel intensity and interpixel distance as its two parameters, as the edge weight between a pair of pixels. Let I_j and I_k be the intensity values of two pixels j and k, and let d_{jk} be the Euclidean distance between them. Then the capacity function c_{jk} is given by

$$c_{jk} = \frac{I_j I_k}{d_{jk}}. \tag{8.3}$$

Since a typical fracture is marked by loss of bone material, the average pixel intensity of a fracture site is lower than that of the surrounding bone. Additionally, the distance between two boundary pixels would be expected to be relatively higher if they straddled a fracture site. Moreover, the influence of tangential neighbors would be expected to be greater than that of the normal neighbors due to the incorporation of the Euclidean distance in the capacity function. This justifies the formulation of the capacity function, as given by (8.3). Very high capacity values are assigned to the edges which connect vertices q_f and r_f to the source vertex s and those which connect the sink vertex t to vertices q_l and r_l. By virtue of its construction, all edges in the proposed flow network have capacity > 0. A schematic diagram of a 2D flow network with the source vertex, sink vertex, tangential edges, and normal edges is shown in Fig. 8.1.

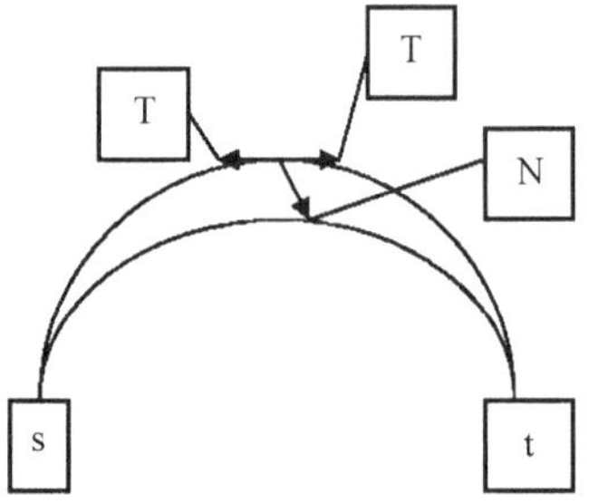

Fig. 8.1 A schematic 2D flow network with a source vertex (s), a sink vertex (t), tangential edges (T), and normal edges (N)

8.4.2 Correctness of the 2D Flow Network Model

The purpose of this subsection is to provide an intuitive justification for the correctness of our modeling of fracture detection as a 2D graph cut. We follow the framework of Boykov and Jolly [150]. Based on its definition, each cut C in the flow network G satisfies the following two properties:

1. C groups the vertices of G into two disjoint sets.
2. One set contains the source vertex s, and the other set contains the sink vertex t.

Claim 8.1 *A minimum cut C^* correctly identifies a fracture in the proposed flow network G.*

Justification The justification is based on Theorem 2.5 and the construction of the proposed flow network based on the capacity function given by (8.3). We seek to determine the maximum flow between s and t. Using Theorem 2.5, we obtain the minimum cut C^* consisting of the minimum-cut edges in the flow network G. Essentially, the minimum-cut edges are edges in the flow network with comparatively low capacity values. From (8.3) it is evident that the low-capacity edges are edges with relatively lower pixel intensity values and relatively higher distance values. These are precisely the characteristics of an edge in the vicinity of a fracture site. Thus, identification of a minimum cut intuitively corresponds to detection of a fracture. □

The computation of the augmenting path in the flow network was done using *breadth-first search*, as outlined in the *Edmonds–Karp* algorithm [35] for determining the max-flow and min-cut in a flow network. The *Edmonds–Karp* algorithm is a variant of the classic *Ford–Fulkerson* algorithm and has a worst-case time-complexity of $O(|V||E|^2)$, where $|V|$ denotes the cardinality of the vertex set V and $|E|$ denotes the cardinality of the edge set E in the flow network G.

8.5 Max-Flow Min-Cut in 3D

In this section we extend the results of the previous section to a 3D scenario. As mentioned earlier, the input to our problem is a 2D CT image sequence of a fractured mandible. We can run the 2D max-flow min-cut algorithm separately for each 2D CT image slice. However, integrating the results from the individual CT image slices is a challenge. Thus, instead of employing the Ford–Fulkerson algorithm on the individual 2D CT image slices, we employ the algorithm on the 3D CT image stack as a whole. This calls for the construction of a 3D flow network for the CT image stack.

8.5.1 Construction of the 3D Flow Network

In a typical CT image stack, the axial resolution (i.e., resolution along the Z axis) of the CT image sequence is much lower than the 2D resolution in the XY plane.

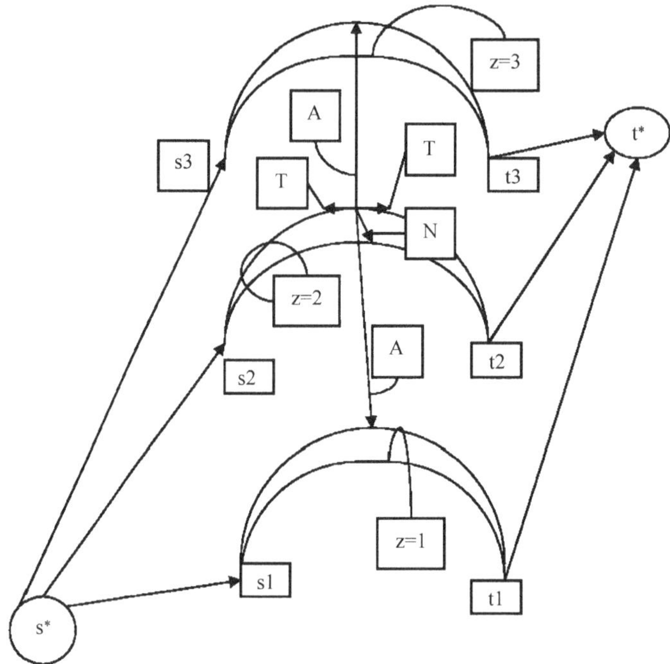

Fig. 8.2 A schematic 3D flow network with a hypersource vertex s^*, a hypersink vertex t^*, source vertices $(s1, s2, s3)$, sink vertices $(t1, t2, t3)$, tangential edges (T), normal edges (N), and axial edges (A)

We use simple volume interpolation along the Z axis to ensure that the voxels are cubic instead of rectangular parallelopipeds. Having uniform resolution along all the three axes renders the setting more amenable for a 3D graph cut. The fractures are observed to occur in approximately the same location in the different CT image slices in which they appear.

For the 3D flow network $G_{3D} = (V_{3D}, E_{3D})$, we add a hypersource vertex s^* below the left condyle in the first CT image slice and a hypersink vertex t^* below the right condyle in the last CT image slice. Thus, the new vertex set can be written as

$$V_{3D} = \{s^*, t^*\} \cup \bigcup_{i \in n_s} V_i,$$

where n_s is the number of CT image slices, and V_i denotes the set of vertices in the ith CT image slice. The set of edges E_{3D} of the 3D flow network are created as follows. We create a set of edges from s^* to source vertices s_i in the individual CT image slices and edges from the sink vertices t_i in the individual CT image slices to t^*. A very high capacity value is assigned to the edges connecting s^* to the s_i's and t_i's to t^*. Axial edges A are constructed between pixels on any two adjacent slices at similar locations (i.e., having the same (x, y) values) in the individual CT image slices. Thus, the edge set E_{3D} is given by

$$E_{3D} = A \cup \bigcup_{i \in n_s} \left(\{ (s_i, s^*), (t_i, t^*) \} \cup E_i \right),$$

where E_i denotes the set of edges in the 2D flow network corresponding to the ith CT image slice. A schematic diagram of a 3D flow network is shown in Fig. 8.2. In this figure, we show a 3D flow network for 3 consecutive CT image slices with a hypersource vertex s^*, hypersink vertex t^*, source vertices s_1, s_2, and s_3, and sink vertices t_1, t_2, and t_3 for the individual 2D CT images slices with axial coordinates $z = 1$, $z = 2$, and $z = 3$, respectively. The tangential (T), normal (N), and axial (A) edges are also shown in Fig. 8.2.

8.5.2 Correctness of the 3D Flow Network Model

Now, we state and justify the following claim for the 3D flow network, which is an extension of the flow network designed for the 2D case:

Claim 8.2 *A minimum cut C^{3D*} in the proposed 3D flow network G_{3D} correctly identifies a fracture.*

Justification Based on Theorem 2.7, the maximum flow problem in a multiple source multiple sink flow network becomes a maximum flow problem in an equivalent graph with a single hypersource and a single hypersink. Our construction of the 3D flow network already satisfies the construction criterion of Theorem 2.7. Subsequently, we can use the same argument used in the justification of Claim 8.1 to complete an intuitive proof for the present claim. □

8.6 Experimental Results

We show the results of the 2D max-flow min-cut algorithm for two different mandibles in Figs. 8.3 and 8.4. In each of these figures, the centers of the crosses mark the source and the sink vertices, and the fractures are indicated by dark squares. After execution of the max-flow min-cut algorithm, we obtain the edges in the cut set. Each such edge joins a vertex on the source-side with another vertex on the sink-side of the flow network. For proper visualization, each such vertex is represented by a black square. The fractures are identified accurately in both the cases.

We conclude this section with an example of a 3D graph cut shown in Fig. 8.5. The hypersource vertex is in the first CT image slice, and the hypersink vertex is in the last CT image slice, and both are marked by large white crosses. The source and the sink vertices in the individual CT image slices are marked by the smaller dark crosses. Once again, the fractures are indicated by dark squares. It is found that running the max-flow min-cut algorithm on a 3D flow network results in better

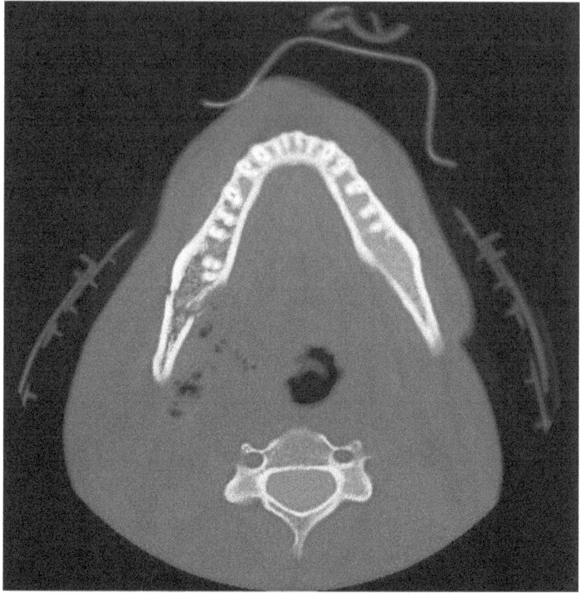

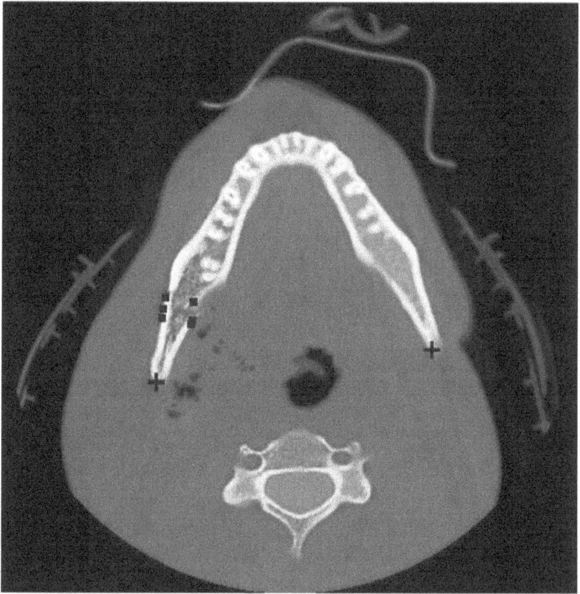

Fig. 8.3 Dataset-I: A fractured mandible is shown on the *top*. The result of fracture detection with the source and sink vertices identified is shown on the *bottom*

visualization of the fractures than running the max-flow min-cut algorithm over the individual 2D image slices. A 3D surface obtained from the above six slices, with fractures detected, is shown in Fig. 8.6. The fractures are indicated by dark squares within a black ellipse. The max-flow min-cut algorithm when run on the 3D flow network corresponding to Fig. 8.5 takes about a minute to complete on a 1.73-GHz Intel Pentium-M© processor. The max-flow min-cut algorithm, when run on the set

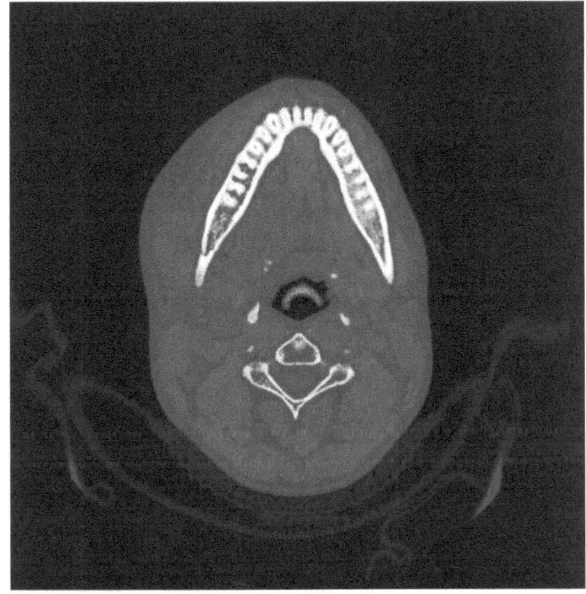

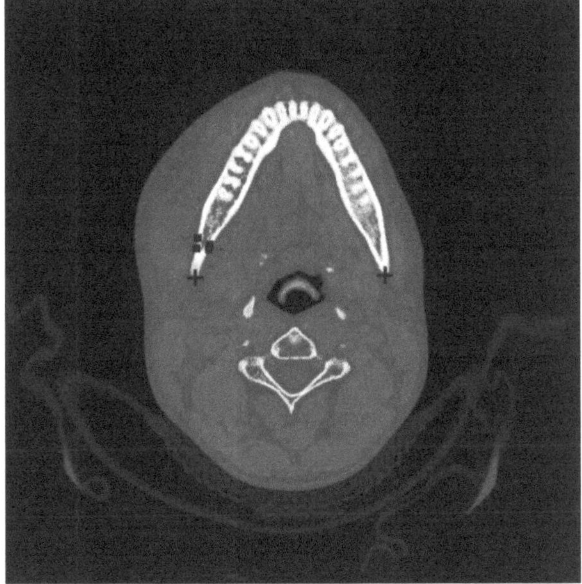

Fig. 8.4 Dataset-II: A fractured mandible is shown on the *top*. The result of fracture detection with the source and sink vertices identified is shown on the *bottom*

of individual 2D flow networks corresponding to the 2D CT image slices in Fig. 8.5, takes a few seconds to complete its execution on the same machine. A surgeon can opt for either a sequence of 2D graph cuts or a single 3D graph cut as the desired outcome based on whether execution time or visualization accuracy is the priority. One can possibly identify the broken fragments by following the augmenting paths in the flow network containing the minimum-cut edges.

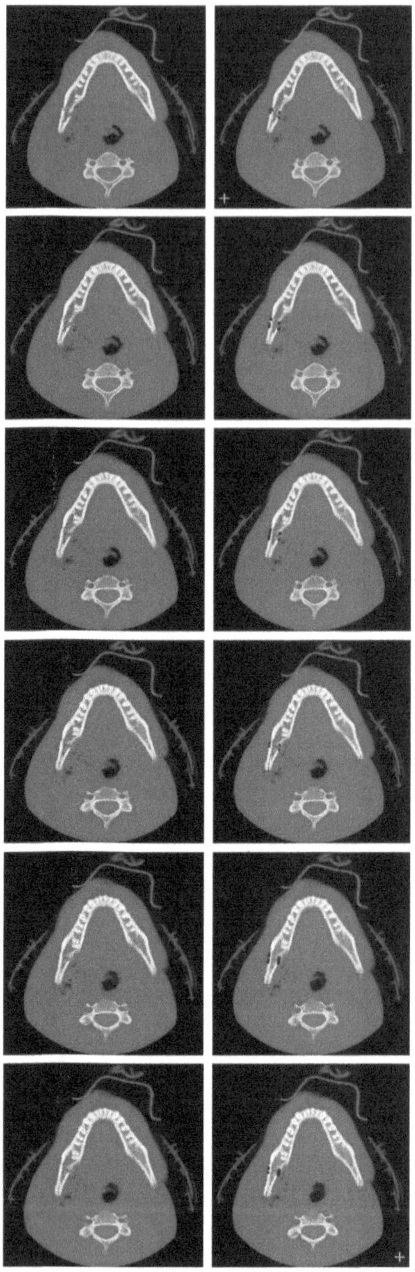

Fig. 8.5 Slicewise mandibular fracture detection using a 3D graph cut. The *first column* shows the input CT image slice. The *second column* shows the output with the source vertices, sink vertices, hypersource vertex, hypersink vertex, and fractures identified

8.7 Conclusion and Future Work

In this chapter, we have presented a novel approach for the detection of mandibular fractures. A fracture is modeled as a minimum cut in a flow network using the well-

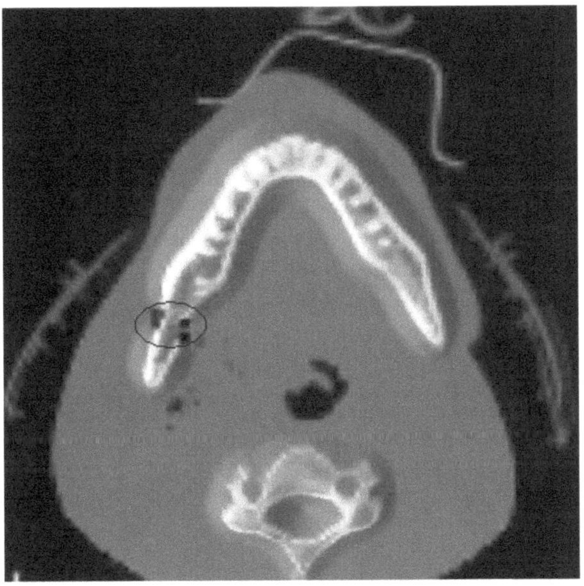

Fig. 8.6 3D surface obtained from the 2D fractured slices, shown in Fig. 8.5. *Black dots* within the ellipse shows the detected fractures

known max-flow min-cut algorithm by Ford and Fulkerson. The method requires no user intervention since the identification of the source vertex, sink vertex, and flow paths in the flow network representation are done automatically. However, the value for the pixel intensity corresponding to the bone material for the purpose of boundary detection is obtained from the domain knowledge. The max-flow min-cut algorithm is used successfully for both 2D flow network and 3D flow network representations. The flow network is constructed based on the knowledge of the geometry of the human mandible and the fracture pattern. Simple capacity functions are designed as edge weights in the flow network representation.

Future work would focus on making the capacity function more robust by incorporation of anatomical knowledge and shape priors [152]. As discussed and shown in the previous chapter, a mandibular fracture is often associated with tissue swelling and presence of certain low-intensity regions called emphysema [146]. One can assign lower weights to the flow network edges in the vicinity of an emphysema and thus make them more likely candidates for a minimum cut. We can add some more normal edges to the flow network representation by examining a small solid angle subtended by a pixel in 2D and by a voxel in 3D. The pixels (or voxels) lying within the solid angle subtended by any pixel (or voxel) can be deemed to be approximate normal neighbors. This would make the resulting flow network more dense and may yield better results. The 2D graph cut algorithm runs very fast (within few seconds), but the 3D graph cut algorithm takes about a minute to execute because of the large size of the 3D flow network. A potential direction for future research would be to use computationally more efficient flow algorithms as those proposed by Boykov and Kolmogorov [156].

Part IV
Concluding Remarks

Chapter 9
GUI Design and Research Synopsis

9.1 Chapter Organization

This chapter presents an overall summary of the research work described in all the previous chapters. We begin the chapter with Sect. 9.2, which describes the design of a Graphical User Interface (GUI). In Sect. 9.3, we provide a synopsis of our research. The synopsis provides a global perspective for our research and emphasizes its interdisciplinary nature. We show how various techniques from graph theory and statistics can be brought to bear on solution of certain critical problems in the realm of virtual craniofacial surgery. In Sect. 9.4, we show that in the process of tackling these critical problems in virtual craniofacial surgery, we have, in fact, addressed some generic and fundamental problems in computer vision and pattern recognition. Finally, in Sect. 9.5, we outline some general problems in the field of virtual craniofacial surgery that need to be tackled in future. Note that each of the previous chapters has concluded with a section outlining future research directions. However, in those sections, we discussed the future work from a relatively narrow perspective of the specific problem being dealt with in that chapter. In contrast, in the final section of this chapter, we provide the reader a more holistic view of future research directions.

9.2 Design of the Graphical User Interface

We have developed a graphical user interface (GUI), which can be used for both surgical training and surgical planning. The GUI provides a means for the surgeon to perform craniofacial reconstruction in an interactive virtual environment (i.e., *in silico*) using CT image data before performing the actual surgery on a real patient. Thus, the GUI enables the fracture detection and virtual reconstruction algorithms to be integrated into an effective (pre)surgical planning tool that can greatly reduce the operative time, cost, risk, and trauma of the actual surgery. The GUI also enables the fracture detection and virtual reconstruction algorithms to be used as a useful

A.S. Chowdhury, S.M. Bhandarkar, *Computer Vision-Guided Virtual Craniofacial Surgery*, Advances in Computer Vision and Pattern Recognition,
DOI 10.1007/978-0-85729-296-4_9,

InSilicoSurgeon 1.0

SINGLE FRAC. RECONS.	DARCES	ICP	Hybrid DARCES_ICP
SINGLE FRAC. RECONS. (Contd.)	Geometric	Hybrid Geometric-ICP	Composite
MULTIPLE FRAC. RECONS.	Build Score	Obtain Pairs	Monitor Reconstruction
FRAC. DETECTION	Bayesian Inference	MRF	Max-Flow Min-Cut
IMAGE PROC.	Simple Thres.	Entropy Thres.	CCL
ACCESSORY MODULE	Display Registered	Surface Data	Volume Data

Fig. 9.1 A snapshot of the GUI of *InSilicoSurgeon*

surgical training tool. The GUI could be used to experiment with and train on different reconstructive surgical techniques on CT image data from real and simulated craniofacial trauma cases in an interactive virtual environment.

The GUI is built on the top of ImageJ, a public-domain Java-based software developed by NIH for performing various image processing tasks [157]. The software package resulting from the integration of the GUI and the fracture detection and virtual reconstruction algorithms is termed as *InSilicoSurgeon* (©University of Georgia Research Foundation, Inc.). Good interface design principles [158] have been followed in the GUI development process. The various fracture detection and virtual reconstruction algorithms discussed previously are embedded in the corresponding buttons of the GUI. Considerable importance has been given to various factors such as the orientation of the buttons, the size of the buttons, and the font size on the titles of the buttons. The use of color in the GUI design is intentionally restricted to gray and black considering the average age of the intended user community, i.e., plastic surgeons in our case.

As mentioned previously, the GUI consists of several buttons. A total of 18 buttons are arranged in 6 rows and 3 columns. A snapshot of the GUI is given in Fig. 9.1.

A brief description of the various buttons in the GUI is as follows:

1. *Single Frac. Recons.*: This and the next GUI topic are devoted to surface matching algorithms for single fracture reconstruction. In particular, this topic consists of the following three buttons:
   (a) *DARCES*: Upon clicking this button, the DARCES algorithm is executed.
   (b) *ICP*: Upon clicking this button, the ICP algorithm is executed.
   (c) *Hybrid DARCES–ICP*: Upon clicking this button, the hybrid DARCES–ICP algorithm is executed.
2. *Single Frac. Recons.* (*Contd.*): This is a continuation of single fracture reconstruction topic. It has the following three buttons:
   (a) *Geometric*: Upon clicking this button, the Geometric algorithm is executed.

   (b) *Hybrid Geometric–ICP*: Upon clicking this button, the hybrid Geometric–ICP algorithm is executed.
   (c) *Composite*: Upon clicking this button, the composite reconstruction procedure, involving surface matching, shape symmetry, and biomechanical stability, is executed.
3. *Multiple Frac. Recons.*: This topic allows a surgeon to perform virtual reconstruction from multiple fractures. The three buttons in this topic perform the following tasks:
   (a) *Build Score*: The scores for the various fracture surfaces are computed, and a score matrix is generated on clicking this button.
   (b) *Obtain Pairs*: Appropriate sets of opposable fracture surface pairs are generated on clicking this button.
   (c) *Monitor Reconstruction*: This button is used to monitor the step-by-step reconstruction of the broken fragments. After each pair of fragments is registered, the user can check the correctness of the reconstruction by clicking this button.
4. *Frac. Detection*: This topic is dedicated to fracture detection The three buttons associated with this topic perform the following functions:
   (a) *Bayesian Inference*: On clicking this button, the stable fracture points in a CT sequence with major or well-displaced fractures are obtained.
   (b) *MRF*: With this button, a user can detect minor or hairline fractures using the MRF-based technique.
   (c) *Max-Flow Min-Cut*: By clicking this button the user can detect minor or hairline fractures using the Ford–Fulkerson Max-Flow Min-Cut algorithm.
5. *Image Proc.*: This topic covers some basic image processing tasks. It consists of the following three buttons:
   (a) *Simple Thres.*: Upon clicking this button, simple thresholding is performed on the input image.
   (b) *Entropy Thres.*: Upon clicking this button, entropy thresholding is performed on the input image.
   (c) *CCL*: Upon clicking this button, the Connected Component Labeling (CCL) algorithm, in conjunction with area based filtering, is executed to complete the segmentation of the bone fragments in the fractured human mandible.
6. *Accessory Module*: This topic serves to provide accessory procedures that are needed at various times during the reconstruction process. The three buttons associated with this topic are:
   (a) *Display Registered*: The broken bone fragments are actually registered and displayed upon clicking this button. For example, when the user clicks on the *ICP* button followed by this button, the broken fragments are registered according to the transformation predicted by the ICP algorithm and subsequently displayed. The same holds for the other surface matching algorithms.
   (b) *Surface Data*: This button enables the user to extract the individual points on the fracture contours. An aggregation or collation of these contour points across multiple CT image slices (in which the fracture is visible) constitutes the surface data that is used for registration or reconstruction.

(c) *Volume Data*: Upon clicking this button, the volume data for a bone fragment is obtained.

9.3 Synopsis

Our monograph altogether consists of four parts including the present one. Part I of the monograph has three chapters. In Chap. 1, we presented the importance of our research in virtual craniofacial surgery. Craniofacial fractures are encountered very frequently in modern society; the principal reasons being gunshot wounds, motor vehicle accidents, and sports-related injuries. We pointed out the paucity of existing work on computer-based automation of detection of craniofacial fractures and reconstruction of the craniofacial skeleton. Our research in virtual craniofacial surgery was motivated by the need to address the following challenges:

1. Computer-aided fracture detection, and
2. Computer-aided virtual craniofacial reconstruction.

We made extensive use of graph theory and statistics in our research. In order to familiarize a general reader with the various techniques from these two disciplines, we included two chapters covering tutorial material. Chapter 2 provided the necessary graph-theoretic foundations. The four sections in Chap. 2 provided the basic terminology in graph theory and covered important graph-theoretic concepts such as graph matching, graph isomorphism, graph automorphism, and network flow. In Chap. 3, we discussed some fundamental statistical concepts. The four sections in Chap. 3 covered the basic concepts underlying probability, statistical inference, Bayesian statistics, and Markov random fields.

Part II of the monograph, which comprises of two chapters, focused on the problem of virtual craniofacial reconstruction. In Chap. 4, we described, in detail, various techniques for single fracture reconstruction. We investigated five different reconstruction algorithms, namely, ICP, DARCES, hybrid DARCES–ICP, Geometric, and hybrid Geometric–ICP. We also employed the theory of fuzzy sets and surface curvature to improve the reconstruction accuracy. Note that the goal thus far was to achieve an accurate matching of the opposing fracture surfaces by minimizing the mean squared surface matching error. We also explored the incorporation of constraints based on anatomical symmetry and biomechanical stability of the human mandible to further improve the reconstruction. We designed a composite reconstruction metric to incorporate the constraints based on bilateral symmetry and biomechanical stability within the reconstruction procedure and proposed an angular perturbation scheme to optimize this metric. Chapter 5 was devoted to the problem of virtual craniofacial reconstruction in the presence of multiple fractures. In the multifracture reconstruction problem, a maximum weight graph matching algorithm was used to identify opposable fracture surfaces in polynomial time. A score matrix based on Hausdorff distance and contour curvature was designed to serve as an input to the graph matching algorithm. A volumetric matching procedure based on the computation of the Tanimoto coefficient was used to monitor the progress of reconstruction at each stage.

Part III of the monograph, which consisted of three chapters, was aimed at computer-aided fracture detection. Both, major or well-displaced fractures and minor or hairline fractures were considered. In Chap. 6, major or well-displaced fractures were detected using a two-step process. In the first step, corner points or points of high curvature were detected as potential fracture points. In the second step, a Kalman filter, implemented within a Bayesian inference paradigm, was used to filter out the spurious corner points and retain the anatomically consistent ones. In Chap. 7, an MRF-based hierarchical Bayesian approach was undertaken for detection of minor or hairline fractures and for target pattern generation. The proposed MRF-based scheme consisted of two steps. In the first step, coarse fracture localization was performed using statistical cross-correlation and by exploiting the bilateral symmetry of the human mandible. Following the approach of Geman and Geman, we modeled the fracture as a stochastic local degradation of a hypothetical intact mandible. In the second step, we estimated the mode of the posterior distribution, which led to the generation of the target pattern, i.e., the reconstructed jaw. The differences in pixel intensity at specific pixel locations between the input CT images and the CT images corresponding to the mode estimate of the posterior distribution were used to localize the hairline or minor fracture. The target pattern was observed to simulate the natural bone healing process and thus had the potential to be used as a prognostic tool. By examining the target pattern a surgeon could decide if open surgical reduction and fixation was necessary or whether the fractures could be managed by allowing them to heal spontaneously. In Chap. 8, we modeled a minor or hairline fracture as a minimum cut in an appropriately weighted flow network representation of the human mandible. We employed the Edmonds–Karp enhanced Ford–Fulkerson algorithm to obtain a minimum cut and thereby detect a minor or hairline fracture.

9.4 Virtual Reconstructive Surgery—An Interdisciplinary Research Perspective

One of the primary motivations of this monograph was to underscore the interdisciplinary nature of the research in virtual reconstructive surgery. We have shown the problems of computer vision-aided fracture detection and computer vision-aided virtual reconstruction to be not only of practical interest to practicing surgeons and radiologists but also of significant theoretical and mathematical interest to researchers in computer vision and pattern recognition community. We have successfully cast the problems of computer vision-aided fracture detection and computer vision-aided virtual reconstruction as well-known problems in two diverse disciplines, i.e., graph theory and statistics. Our investigation of concepts and algorithms from these two diverse disciplines resulted in the following contributions to the research in the general area of computer vision and pattern recognition:

1. Formulation of a hybrid DARCES–ICP algorithm for single-fracture and multi-fracture craniofacial reconstruction. The hybrid algorithm was observed to combine the accuracy of the ICP algorithm with the outlier removal capability of the DARCES algorithm. (Chap. 4)
2. Formulation of a systematic procedure for generation of multiple initial states for the ICP algorithm based on concepts underlying Graph Automorphism. The resulting algorithm, termed as the hybrid Geometric–ICP algorithm, was shown to outperform the conventional ICP algorithm. (Chap. 4)
3. Use of the Maximum Cardinality Minimum Weight Bipartite Graph Matching (MCMW) algorithm to solve the correspondence problem in the ICP algorithm for single-fracture and multifracture craniofacial reconstruction. (Chaps. 4 and 5)
4. Formulation of the 3D jigsaw puzzle problem as a Maximum Weight Graph Matching (MWGM) problem. This was an alternative to the existing formulation of the 3D jigsaw puzzle problem as a Traveling Salesperson Problem (TSP). The resulting MWGM algorithm was observed to have a polynomial worst-case time complexity as opposed to exponential worst-case time complexity of most algorithms that solve the TSP. The solution to the 3D jigsaw puzzle problem was shown to be a precursor to the solution to the multi-fracture craniofacial reconstruction problem. (Chap. 5)
5. Formulation of the problem of detecting stable fracture surface points, in the case of major fractures, as one of specification of a reliable zone for spatial consistency using Bayesian credible sets. (Chap. 6)
6. Formulation of the hairline fracture detection problem as an image restoration problem with a partially unknown local stochastic degradation. Solution to the aforementioned image restoration problem using an MRF-based hierarchical Bayesian approach. Demonstration of the prognostic capability of the generated target pattern for predicting the outcome of natural bone healing. (Chap. 7)
7. Modeling of a fracture, which is essentially a surface discontinuity, as a minimum cut in an appropriately weighted flow network representation of the craniofacial skeleton. Use of the Edmonds–Karp enhanced Ford–Fulkerson algorithm for obtaining a minimum cut leading to the detection of hairline or minor fractures. (Chap. 8)

9.5 Future Research Directions

We have been successful in predicting an accurate 3D rigid body transformation for bringing the broken mandibular bone fragments into registration and thereby reconstructing the fractured craniofacial skeleton. A potential major direction for future work could be the use of a (tele)robotic arm to perform the actual surgery. The surgical procedure, thus automated, could be monitored by an experienced surgeon. Thus, we can substantially increase the degree of automation in the surgical procedure and yet have a surgeon within the loop for overall supervision and intervention in the event of any software or hardware failure. The surgical procedure, thus automated, would allow the surgeon to perform the surgery with greater precision, with fewer and better targeted incisions in significantly less time. Such an automated surgical technique would also entail lower operative costs, less operative and post-operative trauma or risk to the patient, and a faster postoperative recovery for the patient. Another important direction for future research would be the development of an anatomical model of the human craniofacial skeleton and use of the model-guided feedback for further improvement of the overall virtual reconstruction. The formulation of an anatomically and biomechanically accurate model of craniofacial skeleton would also allow the surgeon to design the prostheses in advance of the actual operation. It would also allow the surgeon to verify the design, placement and affixation of the prostheses *in silico* so that the resulting reconstruction is both anatomically correct and biomechanically sound.

We have investigated different techniques for detecting major or well-displaced and minor or hairline fractures. As discussed earlier, the detection of surface points of high curvature, followed by use of the Kalman filter implemented within a Bayesian inference paradigm enables the identification of major or well-displaced fractures. In contrast, the MRF-based hierarchical Bayesian reconstruction scheme and the max-flow min-cut algorithm of Ford and Fulkerson were able to detect minor or hairline fractures. A major challenge is to design a unified scheme for identifying and localizing accurately all types of fractures. Another problem that warrants further investigation is the automatic selection of potential fracture-containing CT image slices from a given CT image sequence (stack). It has been our general observation that in a typical CT image stack consisting of several image slices, the fractured mandible appears in only a few. In the work described in this monograph, we have manually identified, from within the entire CT image stack, the subset(s) of CT image slices that contain the fracture(s). Our fracture detection and reconstruction algorithms were then employed on these select subsets to accurately detect the fractures and reconstruct the mandible, respectively. In order to have a more automated scheme, one could conceivably first employ content-based image retrieval (CBIR) strategies in medical images to identify and isolate the subset(s) of the potential fracture-containing CT image slices [159, 160]. As an example, knowledge of the shape and intensity of the craniofacial skeleton can be used in this particular problem. Once the potential fracture-containing CT image slices are automatically identified within the sequence using suitable CBIR strategies, the proposed fracture detection and virtual reconstruction techniques can be applied on them.

References

1. King RE, Scianna JM, Petruzzelli GJ (2004) Mandible fracture patterns: A suburban trauma center experience. Am J Otolaryngol 25(5):301–307
2. Ogundare BO, Bonnick A, Bayley N (2003) Pattern of mandibular fractures in an urban major trauma center. J Oral Maxillofac Surg 61(6):713–718
3. Zahl C, Muller D, Felder S, Gerlach KL (2003) Cost of miniplate osteosynthesis for treatment of mandibular fractures: a prospective evaluation. Gesundheitswesen 65(10):561–565
4. Pashley DH, Borke JL, Yu JC (2002) Biomechanics and craniofacial morphogenesis. In: Lin KY, Ogle RC, Jane JA (eds) Craniofacial surgery—science and surgical technique. Saunders, Philadelphia
5. Kurihara T (2001) The fourth dimension in simulation surgery for craniofacial surgical procedures. Keio J Med 50(2):155–165
6. Nakajima H, Kaneko T, Kurihara T, Fujino T (2001) Craniofacial surgical simulation in the 3-dimensional CT SurgiPlan system. Keio J Med 50(2):95–102
7. Siessegger M, Schneider BT, Mischkowski RA, Lazar F, Krug B, Klesper B, Zoller JE (2001) Use of an image-guided navigation system in dental implant surgery in anatomically complex operation sites. J Craniomaxillofac Surg 29(5):276–281
8. Eldeeb H, Boubekri N, Asfour S, Khalil T, Finnieston A (2001) Design of thoracolumbosacral orthosis (TLSO) braces using CT/MR. J Comput Assist Tomogr 25(6):963–970
9. Bechtold JE, Powless SH (1993) The application of computer graphics in foot and ankle surgical planning and reconstruction. Clin Podiatr Med Surg 10:551–562
10. Sutherland CJ, Bresina SJ, Gayou DE (1994) Use of general purpose mechanical computer assisted engineering software in orthopaedic surgical planning: advantages and limitations. Comput Med Imaging Graph 18:435–442
11. Chao EYS, Sim FH (1995) Computer-aided preoperative planning in knee osteotomy. Iowa Orthop J 15:4–18
12. Byrd HS, Hobar PC (1993) Rhinoplasty: a practical guide for surgical planning. Plast Reconstr Surg 91:642–654
13. Ayoub AF, Wray D, Moos KF, Siebert P, Jin J, Nibbet TB, Urquhart C, Mowforth P (1996) Three-dimensional modeling for modern diagnosis and planning in maxillofacial surgery. Int J Adult Orthodon Orthognath Surg 11(3):225–233
14. Gerbo LR, Poulton DR, Covell DA, Russell CA (1997) A comparison of a computer-based orthognathic surgery prediction system to postsurgical results. Int J Adult Orthodon Orthognath Surg 12(1):55–63
15. Hassfeld S, Zoller J, Albert FK, Wirtz CR, Knauth M, Muhling J (1998) Preoperative planning and intraoperative navigation in skull base surgery. J Craniomaxillofac Surg 26(4):220–225
16. Patel VV, Vannier MW, Marsh JL, Lo LJ (1996) Assessing craniofacial surgical simulation. IEEE Comput Graph Appl 16(1):46–54

A.S. Chowdhury, S.M. Bhandarkar, *Computer Vision-Guided Virtual Craniofacial Surgery*, Advances in Computer Vision and Pattern Recognition,
DOI 10.1007/978-0-85729-296-4,

17. Verstreken K, Van Cleynenbreugel J, Marchal G, Naert I, Suetens P, van Steenberghe D (1996) Computer-assisted planning of oral implant surgery: A three-dimensional approach. Int J Oral Maxillofac Implants 11(6):806–810
18. Hilger KB, Larsen R, Wrobel MC (2003) Growth modeling of human mandibles using non-Euclidean metrics. Med Image Anal 7(4):425–433
19. Cevidanes LHS, Styner M, Phillips C, Oliveira AEF, Tulloch JFC (2007) 3D morphometric changes 1 year after jaw surgery. In: Proc fourth IEEE symp biomedical imaging (ISBI), pp 1332–1335
20. Enciso R, Memon A, Neumann U, Mah J (2003) The virtual cranio-facial patient project: 3D modelling and animation. In: Westwood JD, Hoffman HM, Mogel GT, Phillips R, Robb RA, Stredney D (eds) Proc eleventh medicine meets virtual reality conf, pp 65–72
21. Mollemans W, Schutyser F, Nadjmi N, Suetens P (2005) Very fast soft tissue predictions with mass tensor model for maxillofacial surgery planning systems. In: Proc ninth annual conf intl soc for comput aided surg, pp 491–496
22. Mandible Reconstruction Project, Imaging Technology Group, University of Illinois, Urbana-Champaign, IL. URL: http://www.itg.uiuc.edu/technology/reconstruction
23. Virtual Reality Surgical Planning for Mandibular Reconstruction, National Biocomputation Center, Stanford University Medical Center, Palo Alto, CA. URL: http://biocomp.stanford.edu/projects/
24. Ahmed MT, Eid AH, Farag AA (2001) 3D reconstruction of the human jaw: a new approach and improvements. In: Proc medical image computing and computer assisted intervention, pp 1007–1014
25. Joskowicz L, Milgrom C, Simkin A, Tockus L, Yaniv Z (1998) FRACAS: a system for computer-aided image-guided long bone fracture surgery. Comput Aided Surg 3(6):271–288
26. Mack MJ (2001) Minimally invasive and robotic surgery. JAMA 285(5):568–572
27. Peters TM (2006) Image-guidance for surgical procedures. Phys Med Biol 51:R505–R540
28. Dimaio SP et al (2006) Image-guided neurosurgery at Brigham and Women's Hospital—the integration of imaging navigation and interventional devices. IEEE Eng Med Biol Mag 25(5):67–73
29. Vosburgh KJ, Jolesz FA (2003) The concept of image-guided therapy. Acad Radiol 10:176–179
30. Sholmovitz E, Amaral JG, Chait PG (2006) Image-guided therapy and minimally invasive surgery in children: a merging future. Pediatr Radiol 36:398–404
31. Papadimitriou CH, Steiglitz K, Combinatorial optimization: algorithms and complexity, Prentice Hall, India, 1982
32. Bollobás B. (1998) Modern graph theory. Springer, New York
33. Christofides N (1975) Graph theory: an algorithmic approach. Academic Press, San Diego
34. Valiente G (2002) Algorithms on trees and graphs. Springer, Berlin–Heidelberg
35. Cormen TH, Leiserson CE, Rivest RL, Stein C (2001) Introduction to algorithms. MIT Press, Cambridge
36. Ford LR Jr, Fulkerson DR (1962) Flows in networks. Princeton University Press, Princeton
37. Miller I, Miller M (1999) John E Freund's mathematical statistics with applications. Prentice Hall, New York
38. Bhattacharyya GK, Johnson RA (1977) Statistical concepts and methods. Wiley, New York
39. Gelman A, Carlin JB, Stern HS, Rubin DB (2000) Bayesian data analysis. Chapman & Hall/CRC, London
40. Li SZ (1995) Markov random field modeling in computer vision. Springer, London
41. Geman S, Geman D (1984) Stochastic relaxation, Gibbs distributions, and the Bayesian restoration of images. IEEE Trans Pattern Anal Mach Intell 6(6):721–741
42. Besag J (1974) Spatial interaction and the statistical analysis of lattice systems (with discussions). J R Stat Soc Ser B 36:192–236
43. Winkler G (2003) Image analysis, random fields and Markov chain Monte Carlo methods. Springer, Berlin–Heidelberg
44. Keeve E, Girod S, Girod B (1996) Craniofacial surgery simulation. In: Proc fourth int conf on visualization in biomedical computing, Hamburg, Germany, pp 541–546

45. Sarti A, Gori R, Marchetti C, Bianchi A, Lamberti C (2000) Maxillofacial virtual surgery from 3D CT images. In: Akay M, Marsh A (eds) VR in medicine. Springer, Berlin
46. Zachow S, Hedge HC, Deuflhard P (2006) Computer assisted planning in cranio-maxillofacial surgery. J Comput Inf Technol Sp Issue Comput-Based Craniofacial Model Reconstr 14(1):53–64
47. Besl PJ, McKay ND (1992) A method for registration of 3-D shapes. IEEE Trans Pattern Anal Mach Intell 14(2):239–256
48. Maintz JBA, Viergever MA (1998) A survey of medical image registration. Med Image Anal 2(1):1–36
49. Granger S, Pennec X, Roche A (2001) Rigid point-surface registration using an EM variant of ICP for computer guided oral implantology. In: Proc int conf on medical image computing and computer assisted intervention (MICCAI), Utrecht, The Netherlands, pp 752–761
50. Chen CS (1999) RANSAC-based DARCES: A new approach to fast automatic registration of partially overlapping range images. IEEE Trans Pattern Anal Mach Intell 21(11):1229–1234
51. Rogers M, Graham J (2002) Robust active shape model search for medical image analysis. In: Proc int conf on medical image understanding and analysis, Portsmouth, UK, pp 1–4
52. Ourselin S, Roche A, Prima S, Ayache N (2000) Block matching: A general framework to improve robustness of rigid registration of medical images. In: Proc third int conf on medical robotics, imaging and computer assisted surgery, Pittsburgh, USA, pp 557–566
53. Bhandarkar SM, Chowdhury AS, Tang Y, Yu JC, Tollner EW (2004) Surface matching algorithms for computer aided reconstructive plastic surgery. In: Proc second IEEE int symp on biomedical imaging (ISBI), Arlington, VA, USA, pp 740–743
54. Bhandarkar SM, Chowdhury AS, Tang Y, Yu JC, Tollner EW (2007) Computer vision guided virtual craniofacial reconstruction. Comput Med Imaging Graph 31(6):418–427
55. Bhandarkar SM, Chowdhury AS, Tollner EW, Yu JC, Ritter EW, Konar A (2005) Surface reconstruction for computer vision-based craniofacial surgery. In: Proc seventh IEEE int workshop on applications of computer vision (WACV), Breckenridge, CO, USA, pp 257–262
56. Chowdhury AS, Bhandarkar SM, Robinson RW, Yu JC (2007) Novel graph theoretic enhancements to ICP-based virtual craniofacial reconstruction. In: Proc fourth IEEE int symp on biomedical imaging (ISBI), Arlington, VA, USA, pp 1136–1139
57. Chowdhury AS, Bhandarkar SM, Robinson RW, Yu JC (2009) Virtual craniofacial reconstruction using computer vision, graph theory and geometric constraints. Pattern Recogn Lett 30(10):931–938
58. Wang Y, Peterson B, Staib L (2000) Shape-based 3D surface correspondence using geodesics and local geometry. In: Proc first IEEE int conf on computer vision and pattern recognition (CVPR), Hilton Head Island, USA, pp 644–651
59. Pohl KM, Warfield SK, Kikinis R, Grimson WEL, Wells WM (2004) Coupling statistical segmentation and PCA shape modeling. In: Proc seventh int conf on medical image computing and computer assisted intervention (MICCAI), Saint Malot, France, pp 151–159
60. Chowdhury AS, Bhandarkar SM, Tollner EW, Zhang G, Yu JC, Ritter E (2005) A novel multifaceted virtual craniofacial surgery scheme using computer vision. In: Liu Y, Jiang T, Zhang C (eds) Proc computer vision for biomedical image applications: current techniques and future trends (CVBIA), an ICCV workshop, Beijing, China. LNCS, vol 3765, pp 146–159
61. Hounsfield GN (1980) Nobel award address: computed medical imaging. Med Phys 7(4):283–290
62. Sahoo PK, Soltani S, Wong KC, Chen YC (1988) A survey of thresholding techniques. Comput Vis Graph Image Process 41:233–260
63. Hamilton WR (1847) On quaternions. Proc R Ir Acad, Sci 3:1–16
64. Rangarajan A, Chui H, Mjolsness E, Pappu S, Davachi L, Goldman-Rakic PS, Duncan JS (1997) A robust point matching algorithm for autoradiograph alignment. Med Image Anal 1(4):379–398
65. Kim W, Kak AC (1991) 3-D object recognition using bipartite matching embedded in discrete relaxation. IEEE Trans Pattern Anal Mach Intell 13(3):224–251

66. Kuhn HW (1955) The Hungarian method for the assignment problem. Nav Res Logist Q 2:83–97
67. Yarger R, Quek F (2000) Surface parameterization in volumetric images for feature classification. In: Proc first IEEE int symp bioinformatics and biomed engr, Arlington, VA, USA, pp 297–304
68. Besl PJ (1986) Surfaces in early range image understanding. PhD dissertation, Dept of Computer Science, Michigan Univ, Ann Arbor, MI, USA
69. Haralick RM (1984) Digital step edges from zero crossing of second directional derivatives. IEEE Trans Pattern Anal Mach Intell 6(1):58–68
70. Faux ID, Pratt MJ (1979) Computational geometry for design and manufacture. Wiley, New York
71. Suk M, Bhandarkar SM (1992) Three-dimensional object recognition from range images. Springer, Berlin
72. Miyajima K, Ralescu A (1994) Spatial organization in 2D segmented images: Representation and recognition of primitive spatial relations. Fuzzy Sets Syst 65:225–236
73. Veltkamp RC, Latecki LJ (2006) Properties and performance of shape similarity measures. In: Proc tenth IFCS int conf on data science and classification, Ljubljana, Slovenia, pp 1–9
74. Huttenlocher DP, Klanderman GA, Rucklidge WJ (1993) Comparing images using the Hausdorff distance. IEEE Trans Pattern Anal Mach Intell 15(9):850–863
75. Zabrodsky H, Peleg S, Avnir D (1995) Symmetry as a continuous feature. IEEE Trans Pattern Anal Mach Intell 17(12):1154–1166
76. Sun C, Sherrah J (1997) 3D symmetry detection using the extended Gaussian image. IEEE Trans Pattern Anal Mach Intell 19(2):164–169
77. Tuzikov AV, Sheynin SA (2002) Symmetry measure computation for convex polyhedra. J Math Imaging Vis 16:41–56
78. Tuzikov A, Colliot O, Bloch I (2002) Brain symmetry plane computation in MR images using inertia axes and optimization. In: Proc sixteenth int conf on pattern recognition (ICPR), Quebec, Canada, pp 10516–10519
79. Goldstein H (1982) Classical mechanics. Addison-Wesley, Reading
80. Press WH, Flannery BP, Teukolsky SA, Vetterling WT (1992) Numerical recipes in C: the art of scientific computing. Cambridge University Press, Cambridge
81. Prima S, Ourselin S, Ayache N (2002) Computation of the mid-sagittal plane in 3D brain images. IEEE Trans Med Imaging 21(2):122–138
82. Ardekani B, Kershaw J, Braun M, Kanno I (1997) Automatic detection of the mid-sagittal plane in 3-D brain images. IEEE Trans Med Imaging 16(6):947–952
83. Gefan S, Fan Y, Bertrand L, Nissanov J (2004) Symmetry-based 3D brain reconstruction. In: Proc second IEEE int symp on biomedical imaging (ISBI), Arlington, VA, pp 744–747
84. Junck L, Moen JG, Hutchins GD, Brown MB, Kuhl DE (1990) Correlation methods for the centering, rotation and alignment of functional brain images. J Nucl Med 31(7):1220–1226
85. Shames IH (1964) Mechanics of deformable solids. Prentice-Hall, Englewood Cliffs
86. Wan FYM (1995) Introduction to the calculus of variations and its applications. Chapman & Hall, London
87. Wolfson H, Schonberg E, Kalvin A, Lamdan Y (1988) Solving jigsaw puzzles by computer. Ann Oper Res 12:51–64
88. Webster RW, LaFollette PS, Stafford RL (1991) Isthmus critical points for solving jigsaw puzzles in computer vision. IEEE Trans Syst Man Cybern 21(5):1271–1278
89. Da Gama Leitao HC, Stolfi J (2002) A multiscale method for the reassembly of two-dimensional fragmented objects. IEEE Trans Pattern Anal Mach Intell 24(9):1239–1251
90. Yao FH, Shao GF (2003) A shape and image merging technique to solve jigsaw puzzles. Pattern Recognit Lett 24(12):1819–1835
91. Goldberg D, Malon C, Bern M (2004) A global approach to automatic solution of jigsaw puzzles. Comput Geom Theory Appl 28(3):165–174
92. Makridis M, Papamarkos N (2006) A new technique for solving a jigsaw puzzle. In: Proc thirteenth IEEE int conf on image processing (ICIP), Atlanta, GA, USA, pp 2001–2004

93. Barequet G, Sharir M (1997) Partial surface and volume matching in three dimensions. IEEE Trans Pattern Anal Mach Intell 19(9):929–948
94. Ucoluk G, Toroslu I (1999) Automatic reconstruction of broken 3D surface objects. Comput Graph 23:573–582
95. Papaionnou G, Karabassi E, Theoharis T (2002) Reconstruction of three-dimensional objects through matching of their parts. IEEE Trans Pattern Anal Mach Intell 24(1):114–124
96. Huang QX, Flory S, Gelfand N, Hofer M, Pottmann H (2006) Reassembling fractured objects by geometric matching. ACM Trans Graph 25(3):569–578
97. Kampel M, Sablantig R (2004) On 3D mosaicing of rotationally symmetric ceramic fragments. In: Proc seventeenth int conf on pattern recognition (ICPR), Cambridge, UK, pp 265–268
98. Willis A, Cooper D (2004) Bayesian assembly of 3D axially symmetric shapes from fragments. In: Proc sixth IEEE int conf on computer vision pattern recognition (CVPR), Washington DC, USA, pp 82–89
99. Chen WY, Hwang WL, Lin TC (2006) Planar-shape prototype generation using a tree-based random greedy algorithm. IEEE Trans Syst Man Cybern (B) 36(3):649–659
100. Carretero JA, Nahon MA (2005) Solving minimum distance problems with convex or concave bodies using combinatorial global optimization algorithms. IEEE Trans Syst Man Cybern (B) 35(6):1144–1155
101. Ruan S, Tu F, Pattipati KR, Patterson-Hine A (2004) On a multimode test sequencing problem. IEEE Trans Syst Man Cybern (B) 34(3):1490–1499
102. Boole JR, Holtel M, Amoroso P, Yore M (2001) 5196 mandible fractures among 4381 active duty army soldiers, 1980 to 1998. Laryngoscope 111(10):1691–1696
103. Clauser L, Galie M, Mandrioli S, Sarti E (2003) Severe panfacial fracture with facial explosion: Integrated and multistaged reconstructive procedures. J Craniofac Surg 14(6):893–898
104. Schettler D, Roosen K, Heesen J, Kalff R (1989) Timing and techniques of reconstruction and stabilization of combined craniofacial injuries. Neurosurg Rev 12(1):94–105
105. Chen CS, Hsieh WT, Chen JH (2004) Panoramic appearance-based recognition of video contents using matching graphs. IEEE Trans Syst Man Cybern (B) 34(1):179–199
106. Chowdhury AS, Bhandarkar SM, Robinson RW, Yu JC (2006) Virtual craniofacial reconstruction from computed tomography image sequences exhibiting multiple fractures. In: Proc thirteenth IEEE int conf on image processing ICIP, Atlanta, GA, USA, pp 1173–1176
107. Chowdhury AS, Bhandarkar SM, Robinson RW, Yu JC (2009) Virtual multi-fracture craniofacial reconstruction using computer vision and graph matching. Comput Med Imaging Graph 33(5):333–342
108. Schwartz JT, Sharir M (1987) Identification of partially obscured objects in two dimensions by matching of noisy characteristic curves. Int J Robot Res 6(2):29–44
109. Wolfson H (1990) On curve matching. IEEE Trans Pattern Anal Mach Intell 12(5):483–489
110. Costa LF, Cesar RM Jr (2000) Shape analysis and classification, theory and practice. CRC Press, Boca Raton
111. Burdea GC, Wolfson HJ (1989) Solving jigsaw puzzles by a robot. IEEE Trans Robot Autom 5(6):752–764
112. Veltkamp RC (2001) Shape matching: Similarity measures and algorithms. In: Proc IEEE int conf on shape modeling & applications, Genova, Italy, pp 188–197
113. Belongie S, Malik J, Puzicha J (2002) Shape matching and object recognition using shape contexts. IEEE Trans Pattern Anal Mach Intell 24(4):509–522
114. Mills EJ, Dean PM (1996) Three-dimensional hydrogen-bond geometry and probability information from a crystal survey. J Comput Aided Mol Des 10(6):607–622
115. Ozanian T, Phillips R (2000) Image analysis for computer-assisted surgery of hip fractures. Med Image Anal 4(2):137–159
116. Yap DWH, Chen Y, Leow WK, Howe TS, Png MA (2004) Detecting femur fractures by texture analysis of trabeculae. In: Proc int conf on pattern recognition (ICPR), Cambridge, UK, pp 730–733

117. Syiam M, El-Aziem MA, El-Mensshawy M (2004) AdAgen: Adaptive interface agent for X-ray fracture detection. In: Proc IEEE int conf on electrical, electronic and computer engineering (ICEEC), Cairo, Egypt, pp 354–357
118. Lum V, Leow W, Chen Y, Howe Y, Png M (2005) Combining classifiers for bone fracture detection in X-ray images. In: Proc int conf on image processing (ICIP), Genoa, Italy, pp 1149–1152
119. Jia Y, Jiang Y (2006) Active contour model with shape constraints for bone fracture detection. In: Proc European conf on colour in graphics, imaging, and vision (CGIV), Leeds, UK, pp 90–95
120. He JC, Leow WK, Howe TS (2007) Hierarchical classifiers for detection of fractures in X-ray images. In: Kropatsch WG, Kampel M, Hanbury A (eds) Proc int conf on computer analysis of images and patterns (CAIP), Vienna, Austria. LNCS, vol 4673. Springer, Berlin, pp 962–969
121. Donnelley M, Knowles G, Hearn T (2008) A CAD system for long-bone segmentation and fracture detection. In: Elmoataz A et al (eds) Proc IAPR int conf on image and signal processing (ICISP), Cherbourg-Octeville, Normandy, France. LNCS, vol 5099. Springer, Berlin, pp 153–162
122. Welch G, Bishop G (2004) An introduction to the Kalman filter. Tech Report, No 95-041, UNC Chapel Hill
123. Meinhold RJ, Singpurwalla ND (1983) Understanding the Kalman filter. Am Stat 37(2):123–127
124. Chowdhury AS, Bhandarkar SM, Datta GS, Yu JC (2006) Automated detection of stable fracture points. In computed tomography image sequences. In: Proc IEEE int symp on biomedical imaging (ISBI), Arlington, VA, USA, pp 1320–1323
125. Jain R, Kasturi R, Schunck BG (1995) Machine vision. McGraw Hill, New York
126. Pena D, Gutman I (1988) Bayesian approach to robustifying the Kalman filter. In: Spall J (ed) Bayesian analysis of time series and dynamic models. Marcel Dekker, New York, pp 227–253
127. Ye JC, Bresler Y, Moulin P (2000) Asymptotic global confidence regions in parametric shape estimation problems. IEEE Trans Inf Theory 46(5):1881–1895
128. Subramanian KR, Brockway JP, Carruthers WB (2004) Interactive detection and visualization of breast lesions from dynamic contrast enhanced MRI volumes. Comput Med Imaging Graph 28(8):435–444
129. Simonson KM, Drescher SM Jr, Tanner FR (2007) A statistics-based approach to binary image registration with uncertainty analysis. IEEE Trans Pattern Anal Mach Intell 29(1):112–125
130. Gelman A, Carlin JB, Stern HS, Rubin DB (2004) Bayesian data analysis. Chapman & Hall/CRC, Boca Raton
131. Neter J, Kutner M, Wasserman W, Nachsteim C (2002) Applied linear statistical models. McGraw Hill, New York
132. Perez P, Vermaak J, Blake A (2004) Data fusion for visual tracking with particles. Proc IEEE 92(3):495–513
133. Berger JO (1985) Statistical decision theory and Bayesian analysis. Springer, New York
134. Harris CJ, Stephens M (1988) A combined corner and edge detector. In: Proc 4th Alvey vision conference, Manchester, UK, pp 147–151
135. Besag J (1986) On the statistical analysis of dirty pictures. J R Stat Soc Ser B 48(3):259–302
136. Lee SJ, Rangarajan A, Gindi G (1995) Bayesian image reconstruction in SPECT using higher order mechanical models as priors. IEEE Trans Med Imaging 14(4):669–680
137. Choi SM, Lee JE, Kim J, Kim MH (1997) Volumetric object reconstruction using the 3-D MRF model-based segmentation. IEEE Trans Med Imaging 16(6):887–892
138. Chan AK, Zheng L (2001) An artificial intelligent algorithm for tumor detection in screening mammogram. IEEE Trans Med Imaging 20(7):559–567
139. Salli E, Aronen HJ, Savolainen S, Korvenoja A, Visa A (2001) Contextual clustering for analysis of functional MRI data. IEEE Trans Med Imaging 20(5):403–414

140. Chen T, Metaxas DN (2004) Markov random field models. In: Yoo TS (ed) Insight into images. AK Peters, Wellesley
141. Richard FJP (2005) A comparative study of Markovian and variational image-matching techniques in application to mammograms. Pattern Recognit Lett 26(12):1819–1829
142. Popa C, Zdunek R (2005) Penalized least-squares image reconstruction for borehole tomography. In: Proc algorithmy, Podbanske, Slovakia, pp 260–269
143. Martin-Fernandez M, Alberola-Lopez C (2005) An approach for contour detection of human kidneys from ultrasound images using Markov random fields and active contours. Med Image Anal 9(1):1–23
144. Raj A, Singh G, Zabih R (2006) MRF's for MRI's: Bayesian reconstruction of MR images via graph cuts. In: Proc IEEE int cof on computer vision pattern recognition (CVPR), New York, NY, USA, pp 1061–1068
145. Chowdhury AS, Bhattacharya A, Bhandarkar SM, Datta GS, Yu JC, Figueroa R (2007) Hairline fracture detection using MRF and Gibbs sampling. In: Proc eighth IEEE int workshop on applications of computer vision (WACV), Austin, TX, USA, p 56
146. Giannoudis PV, Dinopoulos II (2005) Current concepts of the inflammatory response after major trauma: an update. Injury 36(1):229–230
147. Vodovotz Y et al (2006) In silico models of acute inflammation in animals. Shock 26(3):235–244
148. Molina R (1994) On the hierarchical Bayesian approach to image restoration: Applications to astronomical images. IEEE Trans Pattern Anal Mach Intell 16(11):1122–1128
149. Boykov Y, Veksler O, Zabih R (2001) Fast approximate energy minimization via graph cuts. IEEE Trans Pattern Anal Mach Intell 23(11):1222–1239
150. Boykov Y, Jolly MP (2001) Interactive graph cuts for optimal boundary & region segmentation of objects in N-D images. In: Proc IEEE int conf on computer vision (ICCV), Vancouver, Canada, pp 105–112
151. Xu N, Bansal R, Ahuja N (2003) Object segmentation using graph cuts based active contours. In: Proc IEEE int conf on computer vision pattern recognition (CVPR), Madison, WI, USA, pp 46–53
152. Freedman D, Zhang T (2005) Interactive graph cut based segmentation with shape priors. In: Proc IEEE int conf on computer vision pattern recognition (CVPR), San Diego, CA, USA, pp 755–762
153. Funka-Lea G, Boykov Y, Florin C, Jolly MP, Moreau-Gobard R, Ramaraj R, Rinck D (2006) Automatic heart isolation for CT coronary visualization using graph-cuts. In: Proc IEEE int symp on biomedical imaging, Arlington, VA, USA, pp 614–617
154. Song Z, Tustison N, Avants B, Gee J (2006) Adaptive graph cuts with tissue priors for brain MRI segmentation. In: Proc IEEE int symp on biomedical imaging (ISBI), Arlington, VA, USA, pp 762–765
155. Boykov Y, Jolly MP (2006) Graph cuts and efficient N-D image segmentation. Int J Comput Vis 70(2):109–131
156. Boykov Y, Kolmogorov V (2004) Fast approximate energy minimization via graph cuts. IEEE Trans Pattern Anal Mach Intell 26(9):1124–1137
157. Rasband WS (1997–2008) ImageJ, US National Institutes of Health, Bethesda, Maryland, USA, http://rsb.info.nih.gov/ij/
158. Rogers Y, Sharp H, Preece J (2002) Interaction design beyond human–computer interaction. Wiley, New York
159. Müller H, Michoux N, Bandon D, Geissbuhler A (2004) A review of content-based image retrieval systems in medical applications-clinical benefits and future directions. Int J Med Inform 73(1):1–23
160. Lehmann TM, Güld MO, Thies C, Fischer B, Spitzer K, Keysers D, Ney H, Kohnen M, Schubert H, Wein BB (2004) Content-based image retrieval in medical applications. Methods Inf Med 43(4):354–361

Index

A.S. Chowdhury, S.M. Bhandarkar, *Computer Vision-Guided Virtual Craniofacial Surgery*, Advances in Computer Vision and Pattern Recognition,
DOI 10.1007/978-0-85729-296-4, © Springer-Verlag London Limited 2011

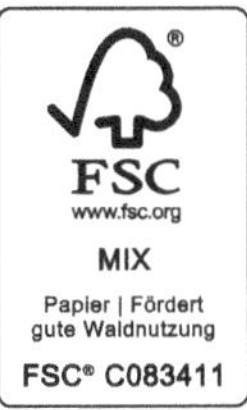

Zeitfracht Medien GmbH
Ferdinand-Jühlke-Straße 7
99095 Erfurt, Deutschland
produktsicherheit@kolibri360.de